2006

I am so amazed with your work ethic! You may be the hardest working student that I have ever encountered! It pays off and you are a perfect example of how dedication leads to success. I was lucky to have you in A+P and AP Biology this year. Keep working hard! Dr. ↓

For Bill

Acknowledgments

Thanks are due to Brandon Toropov, Jen Most, Gigi Ranno, Peter Gouck, Janet Anastasio, Erica Jorgensen, Tami Monahan, and Susan Moffatt for ideas and helpful criticism.

Janet Shoemaker of the American Society for Microbiology, F. Michael Wahl of the Geological Society of America, and Jennie Moehlmann of the American Institute of Biological Sciences were all kind enough to offer advice in selecting the list of women.

The collections of the Boston and Cambridge Public libraries and the Harvard University library system—particularly the Schlesinger Library—were instrumental in the research for this book.

Special thanks go to Cristina Paglinauan, Carolyn Sporn, Rachel Lewis, and my family for their support and aid in research.

Published by Bob Adams, Inc.
260 Center Street, Holbrook, MA 02343

ISBN: 1-55850-361-7

Printed in the United States of America.

J   I   H   G   F   E   D   C   B   A

This book is available at quantity discounts for bulk purchases.
For information, call 1-800-872-5627.

20TH CENTURY WOMEN SERIES

The Remarkable Lives of
100 WOMEN HEALERS and SCIENTISTS

BROOKE BAILEY

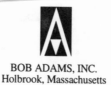

BOB ADAMS, INC.
Holbrook, Massachusetts

Introduction

Women in science have had special obstacles to overcome in the last century. Rules against nepotism blocked some, like psychologists Else Frenkel-Brunswik and Carolyn Wood Sherif, from winning academic posts at the universities that employed their husbands. (The regulations did not, however, prevent those universities from taking advantage of their expertise as untitled instructors.)

For quite some time, women were categorically barred from *enrolling* at some major academic institutions. Such eminent scientists as psychologist Mary Whiton Calkins and astronomer Cecilia Payne-Gaposchkin had to make special arrangements at Harvard University in order to take classes. It seems that many Americans had a hard time imagining why a woman might want to pursue a career in science; one bemused journalist reported on the "spectacle" of biologist Helen Dean King calmly holding a rat in her hand.

Nevertheless, many of the women in this book carved out a space for themselves in fields that were not generally considered "feminine." Some, like Payne-Gaposhkin, managed to balance a traditional home life with their work. Others, like pediatricians Martha May Eliot and Ethel Dunham, created their own nontraditional families.

For many of the women included here, the work alone, regardless of the reward or acknowledgments (or lack thereof), was more fulfilling than any "traditional" choices might have been.

And each woman profiled here handled the choices available to her in a highly personal way. The different paths these women took through often inhospitable circumstances were shaped at least as much by their personalities as by the fields they chose.

The one common element of the stories you're about to read? Every individual included here lived her life fully and on her own terms. And that's worth taking notice of.

— *Brooke Bailey*

Annie Montague Alexander, 1867–1949

A nnie Montague Alexander was a thoroughly original woman who took advantage of a comfortable inheritance to devote her life to the fields of paleontology, botany, ornithology, and mammology. She spent much of her life traveling with her lifetime companion, Louise Kellogg, collecting specimens and enjoying the outdoors. She housed her finds at the museums she founded and funded at the University of California at Berkeley: the Museum of Vertebrate Zoology and the Museum of Paleontology.

Alexander was born in Honolulu, Hawaii, and raised on Maui until the age of fifteen, when the family moved to Oakland, California. Her father made his money investing successfully in real estate; he created a corporation with his partner and brother-in-law Henry Baldwin. Alexander was closest to her father, and after going through the private education and tour of Europe that was expected of genteel young

ladies near the turn of the century, she became his companion on his many trips and tours. This companionship ended sadly on a safari to East Africa, when Alexander's father was killed in a freak accident by a boulder.

On another trip, her interest in the sciences was piqued by her friend Martha Beckwith, an instructor at Mount Holyoke College. "I am beleaguered," Alexander later wrote Beckwith. "What a fever the study of old Earth . . . has set up in me." She began to attend lectures on paleontology at the University of California at Berkeley. By 1903 she was leading expeditions. She became interested in mammals on a series of trips to Alaska and had soon amassed a sizeable collection of skulls of different species. On one trip she found a new subspecies of grizzly bear, which was named *Ursus alexandrae* after her.

In 1909 she collaborated with naturalist Joseph Grinnell to set up the first natural

THE REMARKABLE LIVES OF

history museum on the West Coast. She put up the funds, and he became permanent director of the museum, which was erected on the Berkeley campus out of Alexander's gratitude for her early training there. She also established the university's Department of Paleontology that year. While the museum was being set up, Alexander began taking trips with the woman who would be closest to her for the rest of her life, Louise Kellogg. At the time, Kellogg was twenty-eight; Alexander was forty-one.

From 1911 to 1922, the couple raised cattle and asparagus on their farm on Grizzly Island in the California Suisun Marshes. At fifty-five and forty-three years of age, they returned to the field to go on another long series of collecting trips. Attracted to desert regions, they spent the next fourteen years exploring the deserts of California, Nevada, New Mexico, Utah, Colorado, Idaho, and Arizona. Rough conditions like 136-degree heat and soupy mud did not faze them; they enjoyed eating meals of kangaroo rat ("like chicken," Alexander reported) and sleeping out in the open.

After Joseph Grinnell died in 1939, Alexander and Kellogg turned their attention to botany. They discovered a new, rare species of grass, named *Swallenia alexandrae*, and together they collected over 17,851 botanical specimens for the University of California Herbarium. Their contributions to the Museum of Vertebrate Zoology were equally impressive. Over their lifetime of work together, they contributed specimens of 6,744 different animals to the Museum. Some of these were new to science.

Alexander celebrated her eightieth birthday in Baja California with Kellogg. They continued to take trips into the wild until Alexander suffered a debilitating stroke at eighty-one. She sank into a coma and died several months later. Louise continued to make collecting trips to Baja, but mourned her loss until she died seventeen years later.

> *"What a fever the study of old Earth . . . has set up in me."*

TO FIND OUT MORE . . .

- Bonta, Margaret Meyers. *Women in the Field: America's Pioneering Naturalists.* College Station, TX: Texas A&M University Press, 1991.

- Reifschneider, Olga. *Biographes of Nevada Botanists.* Reno: University of Nevada Press, 1964.

- Alexander's papers are at the Bancroft Library at the University of California at Berkeley. Her field notebooks are at the Museum of Vertebrate Zoology at the University of California at Berkeley.

Hattie Elizabeth Alexander, 1901–1968

Before the bacteriologist and physician's contributions to the battle against influenza meningitis, the disease was always fatal in infants and virtually untreatable in adults. Alexander developed an antiserum that makes deaths from the disease rare today. With the development of the Alexander antibody, **Sarah Elizabeth Branham**'s finding that sulfa drugs could block meningitis, and the later development of penicillin and other antibiotics, virtually the only fatalities from the disease today are in cases that go untreated.

Alexander was a bright girl in a Baltimore family of eight children. She won a scholarship to Goucher College but was a fairly average student there. Her college years didn't hurt her career; she spent three years after college working at the Maryland and U.S. Public Health Services, where she first became interested in bacteriology. Her work there impressed the admissions committee at Johns Hopkins Medical School,

and she was offered a position in the next year's entering class.

If she was an indifferent student in college, at Johns Hopkins she was an ardent one. Her impressive record there and her work in bacteriology earned her an internship at Columbia-Presbyterian Medical Center Babies' Hospital, where she would work with an immunochemist, Dr. Michael Heidelberger. Meningococcal disease was so common at the time that Alexander came into almost daily contact with children dying of the infection. Meningitis attacks the membranes surrounding the brain and spinal cord, sometimes killing its victims within ten hours of the onset of symptoms.

Together, she and Dr. Heidelberger began work on finding a cure for it. It took several years, but eventually, using her background as a bacteriologist, she was able to isolate the meningococcus antibody and formulate an antiserum. The discovery gained her an international reputation; she went on to head the Columbia-Presbyterian Medical Center's microbiological laboratory and the American Pediatrics Society.

Alexander's meningitis antiserum made her famous, but her other contributions to her field, both as a researcher and an instructor, are also significant. She went on to conduct research in bacterial genetics that made her one of the earliest to demonstrate the validity of a theory, then new and unproved, that explicitly linked DNA with genetic characteristics. She was said to be an idiosyncratic teacher who disliked lectures but was intensely focused on her students, drawing them out and inspiring them. Her early death in 1968 was felt as a considerable loss.

> *Alexander's meningitis antiserum made her famous, but her other contributions to her field are also significant.*

TO FIND OUT MORE . . .

- Obituary. *The New York Times*, June 25, 1968.

- Sicherman, Barbara, and Carol Hurd Green, eds. *Notable American Women: The Modern Period. A Biographical Dictionary*. Cambridge, MA: The Belknap Press of Harvard University Press, 1980.

- Vare, Ethlie Ann, and Greg Ptacek. *Mothers of Invention: From the Bra to the Bomb, Forgotten Women and Their Unforgettable Ideas*. New York: William Morrow, 1988.

Elda Emma Anderson, 1899–1961

Elda Anderson was a physicist on the Manhattan Project team, the group that developed the atomic bomb in 1945. She was one of the early health physicists, specialists who work to develop ways of protecting people and the environment from the effects of ionizing radiation. She devoted her life to promoting her budding field, which emerged in the mid-1940s with the growing body of knowledge about the effects of radiation. Her devotion to her work may have contributed to her bouts of leukemia and breast cancer, which plagued her from age fifty-seven until her death at sixty-one.

Lena and Edwin A. Anderson had three children, of whom Elda was the second. As an infant, Edwin had been left on a doorstep in Green Lake, Wisconsin; he grew up to become a mortician and automobile dealer there. Lena had emigrated from Germany to Wisconsin with her parents at age six. Numbers held an early fascination for Elda, who decided on a career in science. Her family, respectful of her evident intellectual ability, supported her ambition. She graduated from Ripon College in 1922 and earned an A.M. in physics from the University of Wisconsin in 1924, with the help of a graduate assistantship.

Elda Anderson became the dean of mathematics and physics at Estherville Junior College in Iowa in 1924, holding the post for three years; there she taught physics, math, and chemistry. She then moved to a two-year stint teaching science at Menasha High School in Wisconsin, and from there to Milwaukee-Downer College. In Milwaukee she was promoted from professor of physics to the chair of the department in 1934. She spent fourteen years with the physics department.

On sabbatical in 1941, Anderson spent some time at Princeton University. The office for which she worked, the Office of Scientific Research and Development, was involved in the beginnings of the Manhattan Project. She left Milwaukee in 1943 to work with the secret group in Los Alamos, New Mexico.

Anderson worked with the other scientists in the group focusing on the cyclotron, a particle accelerator. Her work was relevant both to the development of the bomb and in the design of nuclear reactors. The pace was frantic at Los Alamos; eighteen-hour work days were common, and pressure to produce was high. Anderson adjusted to the pace and stayed for four years, during which she saw the first atom bomb explosion in the desert in 1945 and the end of the war soon afterward. In 1947 she returned to Milwaukee to her old position in the physics department.

Her intense years at Los Alamos had left Anderson with a love of the cutting edge of science, and the quiet academic environment no longer suited her. In 1949, she moved to Tennessee, where she became the Oak Ridge National Laboratory's first chief of education and training in the new Health Physics Division. Until she died in 1961, Anderson worked to make her field recognized as a profession. She established programs in the United States and abroad

Anderson developed ways of protecting people and the environment from the effects of radiation.

and served as secretary pro tem, charter secretary, and president of the Health Physics Society (established by her students).

In 1956, Elda Anderson developed leukemia. She continued her work in her field until her death from breast cancer in 1961. Her students and colleagues at the Health Physics society honored her memory by creating an annual award in her name for the year's outstanding health physicist.

TO FIND OUT MORE . . .

- Obituary. *Health Physics* 5 (1960): 244.

- *The National Cyclopedia of American Biolgraphy* L, pp. 281–2. New York: J.T. White.

- Sicherman, Barbara, and Carol Hurd Green, eds. *Notable American Women: The Modern Period. A Biographical Dictionary.* Cambridge, MA: The Belknap Press of Harvard University Press, 1980.

Virginia Apgar, 1909–1974

Virginia Apgar, a surgeon and anesthesiologist, was one of the first woman surgeons. She switched to anesthesiology, however, when she ran into rigid sexism in surgery. "Women won't go to a woman surgeon . . . only the Lord can answer that one," she said. She is best known for devising the standard Newborn Scoring System, better known as the Apgar score, for evaluating general health in a newborn within one minute of birth.

Apgar was one of the first women to graduate from Columbia University's medical school. She had excelled there, and continued her surgical training with a coveted internship at Columbia-Presbyterian Medical Center. But after two years of successfully performing operations at Columbia-Presbyterian, she came to the disappointing conclusion that she would never be able to make full use of her abilities as a surgeon because of gender bias. She shifted her attention to anesthesiology.

When Apgar began to work in the field, it was mostly populated by nurses and badly needed more scientifically trained specialists. As a female-dominated field, it was often overlooked as a separate medical discipline. Apagar's credentials helped lend weight to her field, and as the director of anesthesiology at Columbia-Presbyterian, she was able to establish it as an entirely new academic department. After eleven years at the head of the department, Columbia made her the first full professor of anesthesiology ever. It was the first time that anesthesiology had been recognized as a medical discipline.

Apgar combined her duties as an administrator with a full load of research, exploring anesthesia and childbirth. In the early 1950s, many newborns were lost to treatable respiratory and circulatory problems. Examinations were conducted long after early treatment could help, in the nursery; at birth the babies were simply swaddled warmly and set aside. Unless the trauma was obvious, it was often overlooked. Apgar, who had attended over seventeen thousand births, introduced her drill in 1952. The Newborn Scoring System ensures that correctable problems don't go unnoticed. It takes a quick measure of pulse, respiration, muscle tone, color, and reflexes.

The "Apgar score" was adopted all over the world, making her internationally famous. She published a book, *Is My Baby All Right?* and was asked to become the director of research of the National Foundation—March of Dimes. While there she made important contributions to the prevention of birth defects and more than doubled the organization's yearly income. She died at 65, still active in her research.

> *Apgar decided to pursue anesthesiology after deciding that gender bias would prevent her from making full use of her skill as a surgeon.*

TO FIND OUT MORE . . .

- Macksey, Joan, and Kenneth Macksey. *The Book of Women's Achievements.* New York: Stein and Day, 1975.

- Vare, Ethlie Ann, and Greg Ptacek. *Mothers of Invention: From the Bra to the Bomb, Forgotten Women and Their Unforgettable Ideas.* New York: William Morrow, 1988.

Sara Josephine Baker, 1873–1945

Physician Sara Baker was one of the pioneering public health administrators who began to shift medical attention to preventative medicine. Her work in the poor areas of New York City, then teeming with infectious diseases, helped to drastically reduce the mortality rates of children under the age of five, who accounted for one-third of all deaths in the city around 1905. As a pioneer in public health, she met with resistance from some fellow physicians, who sent a petition to the Mayor protesting Baker's work because it "was ruining medical practice by its results in keeping babies well." Baker responded with a letter of her own: "This is the first compliment I've had since the Bureau of Child Hygiene was established. I am profoundly grateful for having seen it."

Sara Josephine Baker was one of four children born to a comfortable family in Poughkeepsie, New York. She was the only one of the four who lived to adulthood. Around her graduation from finishing school in her teens, her father died of typhoid fever, leaving her family in dire finan-cial straits. Baker dropped her plans to attend Vassar for the more practical idea of medical school, and by eighteen had passed the entrance requirements for the Women's Medical College of the New York Infirmary for Women and Children in New York City.

At the Women's College, Baker met Florence M. Laighton, with whom she later spent many years practicing medicine and sharing a home. After graduation in 1898, the two spent a year interning together in Boston's New England Hospital for Women and Children. Baker's work there often involved house calls in the poorest neighborhoods, where she once knocked a patient's drunk, belligerent husband down a flight of stairs. In 1899, the two physicians moved back to Manhattan and set up a small private practice, which they ran together until 1914.

Baker began to work for New York City as a medical inspector. She spent seven years in New York slums, trying to save mostly dying children in filthy conditions. In 1907, she captured "Typhoid Mary" Mallon, the cook who had infected seven families with deadly typhoid fever but seemed immune to it herself. Several policemen helped Baker forcibly apprehend Mallon, who was extremely uncooperative at the prospect of having blood drawn.*

As an inspector, Baker found widespread ignorance about hygiene, which she considered the root of many of the city's children's medical problems. During World War I, she liked to say that "it's six times safer to be a soldier in the trenches than to be a baby in the United States."The annual death count dropped by 1,200 in one of her districts in 1908, thanks to her innovative work with a new force of nurses, who sent infected children home from school and taught new mothers basic infant care.

> *Her fellow physicians actually circulated a petition protesting Baker's lowering of infant mortality rates.*

As Baker's success in bringing New York's grim child health statistics under control grew, so did her eminence. She was asked to lecture at NYU's Medical School in 1916, and accepted on the (much protested) condition that she be allowed to enroll in the Doctor of Public Health degree program herself. She earned her degree in 1917.

A lifelong activist, Baker headed sixteen boards of child welfare organizations. From 1935-6, she served as the president of the American Medical Women's Association. She also published a number of authoritative books on child care, including *Healthy Babies* (1920), *Healthy Mothers* (1920), *Healthy Children* (1920), *The Growing Child* (1923), *Child Hygiene* (1925), *Fighting for Life* (autobiography, 1939). Her final years were spent at her home in Trevenna Farm in NJ. At Baker's death at age 75, the New York Times announced that New York had become one of the safest cities in the U.S. for a baby to be born.

TO FIND OUT MORE . . .

- Baker, S. Josephine. *Fighting for Life.* Huntingdon, NY: R.E. Kreiger Pub. Co., 1939.

- O'Hern, Elizabeth Moot. *Profiles of Pioneer Women Scientists.* New York: Acropolis Books, 1985.

- Sicherman, Barbara, and Carol Hurd Green, eds. *Notable American Women: The Modern Period. A Biographical Dictionary.* Cambridge, MA: The Belknap Press of Harvard University Press, 1980.

*Mary Mallon was released two years later, after all efforts to kill the bacteria she carried had failed. She was released on the condition that she return regularly for testing and find work other than cooking, but she broke her promise. She turned up five years later as the source of more infections, and lived the rest of her life confined to North Brother Island.

Florence Bascom, 1862–1945

Geologist Florence Bascom had a string of impressive "firsts" on her way to a successful career: She was the first woman awarded a Ph.D. by Johns Hopkins, she was the first woman elected a fellow of the Geological Society of America, and she was the first woman hired by the United States Geological Survey as an assistant geologist. She probably had the most impact on her field, however, with another "first": she established a new geology department at Bryn Mawr College and oversaw it for the next three decades.

Bascom's family was undoubtedly an influence in her choice of an unorthodox career. She was the youngest of three children by her father's second wife. Born in Williamstown, Massachusetts, where her father taught at Williams College, Bascom absorbed his liberal attitude toward education for women. Although women's education was not universally accepted in the 1860s and 1870s, John Bascom believed that it should be promoted equally with men's education.

The family moved to Madison, Wisconsin, when John Bascom took a position as the president of the University of Wisconsin. Three years later, when she was fifteen, Florence enrolled as a freshman at Wisconsin. Although the university had begun to accept women as full-status students five years earlier, the genders were still largely segregated. Men and women used the library at different times, and women were not allowed to attend lectures that were already full of their male peers. Still, Bascom excelled at the University, graduating with a bachelor's degree in Arts and another in Letters in 1882, and earning a third bachelor's degree in Science in 1884.

Bascom stayed on at Wisconsin, which had excellent resources in geology, for her master's degree. She focused her attention on petrography, the classification and description of rocks. The degree was awarded her in 1887. In 1893, she earned her Ph.D. from Johns Hopkins, even though she had been forced to attend as an informal student and the university had never before awarded the degree to a woman. In 1895 she landed at Bryn Mawr as a reader, beginning her long and influential career there.

Over the next ten years she was gradually recognized as an important asset to the school. When she arrived, there was no geology department. Biology, chemistry, and physics had the run of the science building, and Bascom was forced to work out of a makeshift laboratory in storage space. Worse, the president who hired her had been interested in creating a geology department, but his successor, M. Carey Thomas, was not.

Bascom single-handedly carved out some space for her science nevertheless, conducting her own research while giving popular classes and acquiring necessary specimens and equipment. Although she had more than enough students who wanted to major in geology, President Thomas decided in 1899 to make her subject an elective. Bascom countered by handing in her resignation. Faced with the possibility of losing their popular lecturer, the College's trustees reversed the president's decision.

In 1906 Bascom was made a full professor. She spent the school year leading her nationally known department and her summers investigating rock formations in the Mid-Atlantic Piedmont range or relaxing on her farm in western Massachusetts. She was active in numerous geological organizations and publications, and eventually served as vice-president of the Geological Society of America in 1930. She had intended eventually to retire to Massachusetts, but her work occupied her until her death at age eighty-two.

> **Bascom was the first woman to earn a Ph.D. from Johns Hopkins.**

TO FIND OUT MORE . . .

- Arnold, Lois. *Four Lives in Science: Women's Education in the Nineteenth Century.* New York: Schocken Books.

- Sicherman, Barbara, and Carol Hurd Green, eds. *Notable American Women: The Modern Period. A Biographical Dictionary.* Cambridge, MA: The Belknap Press of Harvard University Press, 1980.

- Bascom's papers are in the Sophia Smith collection at Smith College.

Mary Elizabeth Bass, 1876–1956

. . . .

Mary Elizabeth Bass, a pioneering woman physician, spent much of her time working for the advancement of women in medicine. After her formal retirement from a professorship at Tulane University in 1941, she became an important chronicler of the history of women physicians in America, amassing a collection of over 290 monographs and 1,400 pictures and clippings, now kept at Tulane.

She grew up in Carley, Marion County, Mississippi, the second of eight children born to Baptists Mary Eliza Wilkes Bass and Issac Esau Bass, who ran a dry goods store and a mill. Mary attended local schools and went on to earn teaching certificates. She taught for much of her early twenties in Mississippi and Texas public schools.

Her older brother Charles graduated from the Tulane School of Medicine in 1899, and he backed up both Mary and her younger sister Cora when they were inspired to study medicine. Southern medical schools did not accept women students in 1900, so both entered medical school that year at the Woman's Medical College of Pennsylvania. When they graduated in 1904, however, nothing barred them from setting up a private practice in the South, and they both moved to New Orleans, where they practiced medicine near their brother Charles.

There were more barriers to be overcome, however. Women were not then permitted to practice in the hospitals or clinics of New Orleans. Bass fought the restriction by founding, with five other women physicians, a free dispensary for women and children. In 1908 it was established as the New Orleans Hospital for Women and Children (later renamed the Sara Mayo Hospital). Three years later, Bass was one of the first two women appointed to the faculty at Tulane University's School of Medicine.

The position was not a paid one, but within three years she had been promoted to the salaried rank of instructor in clinical medicine. As a member of the Equal Rights Association of New Orleans, Bass was active in lobbying for women's rights. Her presence at Tulane may have contributed in some small way to the university's decision to begin to accept women medical students in 1914. Her long career in New Orleans medicine would be characterized by this split between work for the University and work for women.

At Tulane, Bass taught bacteriology, pathology, and clinical medicine and was a friend and constant mentor to her women students. She did not limit her student friendships to the classroom, and sometimes helped out with advice or money. She was promoted to full professor in 1920. Meanwhile, she was very active in medical organizations locally and nationally. She was the vice-president of the Orleans Parish Medical Society (1923), twice the president of the Women Physicians of the Southern Medical Association (1925–1927), and the fifth president of the Medical Women's National Association (1921–1922). She also served as a delegate to many international conferences.

It was after her retirement from Tulane in 1941 that she made what is perhaps her most lasting contribution. She began to collect the thousands of documents that make up the Elizabeth Bass Collection at Tulane University. Her research provided the background for a column she wrote in the *Journal of the American Women's Medical Association* from 1946 to 1956. "These Were the First" chronicled the careers of early women physicians.

Bass retired from medicine in 1949 to stay with her ailing mother in Lumberton, Mississippi. She never fully withdrew from the medical community, and she was honored after her retirement with the Elizabeth Blackwell Centennial Medal Award in 1953. After Bass died in 1956, a fund for providing student loans to young women was established in her name at Tulane School of Medicine.

> *Bass was an important chronicler of the history of women physicians in America, amassing a collection of over 290 monographs and 1,400 pictures and clippings at Tulane.*

TO FIND OUT MORE . . .

- Sicherman, Barbara and Carol Hurd Green, eds. *Notable American Women: The Modern Period. A Biographical Dictionary.* Cambridge, MA: The Belknap Press of Harvard University Press, 1980.

- Bass's papers are in the Elizabeth Bass Collection on Women in Medicine at Tulane University's Matas Medical Library, and at the Sophia Smith Collection at Smith College.

Ruth Fulton Benedict, 1887–1948

· ·

As one of America's first professional female anthropologists, Ruth Fulton Benedict helped establish her relatively new and esoteric field as central to our understanding of ourselves. As a social scientist, she argued that patterns of behavior and types of personalities are determined by culture, not by race. The concept was a much more radical one in the pre-World War II era, before the sobering reality of the racism that spawned the Nazi concentration camps.

Ruth Fulton was born on June 5, 1887, in a small farming community in the Shenango Valley of upstate New York. Only two years later, her father, a promising young surgeon and researcher, died of an undiagnosed illness. Ruth and her younger sister were raised mostly on their grandparents' farm, although their resourceful mother sometimes moved them with her to jobs teaching and working as a librarian in Missouri and Minnesota. Despite the basic solidity of her family, Fulton had a difficult childhood. An early illness left her with partial deafness, which adults mistakenly interpreted as unresponsiveness. Her father's death left deep marks, and she turned inward, reading the Bible avidly and keeping a journal. Later she would write beautiful introspective poems.

She studied at Columbia Univeristy with such luminaries as Franz Boas, one of the pioneers of anthropology in America, and **Elsie Parsons**. She earned her Ph.D. in 1923 at age 36, and stayed on at Columbia to teach. As a student she wore the same hat and dress week after week, arguing that men often did so—why shouldn't women? Her self-effacing manner and shy stammer could make her seem awkward, but contemporaries like Margaret Mead remembered her with warmth as a passionate anthropologist. Said Mead, "Ruth Benedict's enthusiasm for the anthropological world she had so recently entered and her delight in the detail of primitive ritual and poetry . . . captivated all of us."

In 1934, Benedict published her most influential book, *Patterns of Culture*. In it, she identified different cultural psychological "types," which she labeled Appollonian and Dionysian. The book sent ripples through the field of anthropology, spawning the "culture and personality" movement within the field. The movement explored the links between the cultural forms of a society and the personalities of the individuals who live within it. The book also had an impact outside of scientific circles; its beautifully clear writing helped bring it to the layman's attention. It helped to legitimize anthropology in the public eye.

Benedict's other important work had an even more significant impact on the reading public. *The Crysanthemum and the Sword* (1946) explained, in Benedict's compelling prose, Japanese culture to uneasy Americans. The book was published the year after America's internment camps for Japanese-Americans were closed. It was an important work for anthropologists, but its impact on the general public, who considered Japanese motivations unfathomable and inhuman, was far greater. Benedict made the enemy a little more human.

Benedict had an eye for the big picture; she grappled with enormous questions, spanning all human experience. "The trouble with life," she wrote in her journal, "isn't that there is no answer, it's that there are so many answers." She was remarkable in her ability to synthesize her many answers into a form comprehensible not only to her peers but to the layman. Her intense love of her field still comes across in her books, which are still assigned to beginning anthropology students. Her death at sixty-one cut her work off unexpectedly early.

> **Benedict argued that culture, not race, was the dominant force in determining human behavior patterns.**

TO FIND OUT MORE . . .

- Caffrey, Margaret M. *Ruth Benedict: Stranger in This Land.* Austin, TX: University of Texas Press, 1989.

- Mead, Margaret. *Ruth Benedict.* New York: Columbia University Press, 1974.

- Modell, Judith Schachter. *Ruth Benedict: Patterns of a Life.* Philadelphia: University of Pennsylvania Press, 1983.

Florence Aby Blanchfield, 1882-1971

. . . .

Nurse Florence Aby Blanchfield worked tirelessly to win full army rank for nurses. She joined and quickly worked her way through the ranks of the Army Nurse Corps, becoming the organization's superintendent in 1943. In 1947, she became the first woman to receive a regular commission in the United States Army.

Florence was born in Front Royal, Virginia, and grew up in Oranda, Virginia, one of eight children born to Mary Louvenia Anderson Blanchfield and Joseph Plunkett Blanchfield. Mary Blanchfield was a nurse who came from a long line of doctors, and Joseph Blanchfield was a stonemason. One of Florence's favorite brothers died when she was still young, reinforcing her drive to become a nurse. In fact, all the Blanchfield daughters became nurses. Florence moved to Pittsburgh, Pennsylvania, to attend South Side Hospital Training School for Nurses, graduating at age twenty-four.

She worked as a private-duty nurse for a time before taking positions at hospitals in Bellevue and Pittsburgh, where she supervised other nurses. She also worked at Ancon Hospital in the Panama Canal Zone before joining the Army Nurse Corps (ANC) in 1917. She spent World War I in France, tending wounded soldiers under the orders of regular army officers who knew little about medicine.

Blanchfield returned briefly to her old position at the hospital in Bellevue after the war, but soon returned to the ANC to serve wherever needed. It turned out that she was needed, over the next fifteen years, in Michigan, California, Georgia, Indiana, China, the Philippines, and Washington, D.C. She served on the Surgeon General's staff in Washington in 1935. In 1942, she was promoted to lieutenant colonel in the ANC, and a year later she was made full colonel and the ANC's superintendent.

Although she herself had reached a high rank in the ANC, Blanchfield would not be satisfied until women were able to serve in the army. She worked within the bounds of the ANC to propel nurses into the thick of the military, training them in military regulations and assigning them to front-line stations where they could assist in surgery. She regularly toured combat sites for ideas. In 1945, the Army awarded her the Distinguished Service Medal for her "devotion to duty."

Blanchfield also worked outside the ANC to secure military rank for nurses. Congresswoman Frances Payne Bolton was an ally, and in 1947 the Army-Navy Nurse Act was passed, granting nurses full status. Florence Blanchfield received the first commission ever awarded to a woman in the U.S. Army. She retired soon afterward to collaborate with Mary W. Standlee on a history of the ANC.

Blanchfield lived in Washington, D.C., with her sister and brother-in-law. She continued to receive honors long after her retirement. In 1951 the International Red Cross awarded her the Florence Nightingale Medal. And seven years after her death at the age of eighty-nine, the United States Army hospital in Fort Campbell, Kentucky, was named after her.

> *Blanchfield worked outside the Army Nurse Corps to secure military rank for nurses.*

TO FIND OUT MORE . . .

- Aynes, Edith A. *From Nightingale to Eagle: An Army Nurse's History*. Englewood Cliffs, NJ: Prentice-Hall, 1973.

- Sicherman, Barbara, and Carol Hurd Green, eds. *Notable American Women: The Modern Period. A Biographical Dictionary*. Cambridge, MA: The Belknap Press of Harvard University Press, 1980.

- Blanchfield's papers are in the Col. Florence A. Blanchfield Collection, in the Nursing Archives at Boston University's Mugar Library.

Katherine Burr Blodgett, 1898–1979

R esearch physicist Katherine Blodgett developed "invisible," or nonreflecting, glass in 1938. The glass is widely used in camera lenses and frames for valuable pictures. Since it does not reflect or absorb light, it doesn't interfere with a viewer's enjoyment of a painting or with photographic film's ability to pick up an image. Her invention also made it possible to measure extremely small gradations in thickness of transparent or semitransparent materials—almost down to the molecule.

Katherine's father, a patent attorney for General Electric in Schenectady, New York, died a few weeks before her birth. Her mother moved her children to first France and then Germany so that they would have a chance to learn languages when they were still very young. Blodgett entered American schools at the age of eight and excelled, winning a scholarship to Bryn Mawr College. She set her sights on her father's employer, General Electric, and earned her master's degree at the University of Chicago in order to secure a position there as a laboratory assistant for Dr. Irving Langmuir. In 1926, she supplemented her master's degree by becoming the first woman ever to earn a Ph.D. in physics from Cambridge University. Degree in hand, she returned to Langmuir's laboratory at General Electric.

Fifteen years before, Langmuir had developed an oily substance with the fascinating characteristic of forming a perfect, one-molecule-thick film on the surface of water. Blodgett began to work with the liquid, for which no one had yet been able to develop any practical use. She found that the solution also formed a film one molecule thick on the surface of a metal plate dipped into it. When she tried immersing the plate a second time, another one-molecule-thick layer formed on top of the first. For the first time, it was possible to layer molecules on top of one another, one layer at a time.

The film did even more interesting things to plates of clear glass. Untreated glass lets most light through, so it's possible to see through it easily. It does, however, reflect about one tenth of the light, causing it to have a slightly distorting effect when used in photographic lenses. When Blodgett experimented with different thicknesses of the film on glass, she found that it was possible to eliminate reflection from the glass, rendering it "invisible"—and perfectly unobtrusive.

Blodgett was the first woman to earn a Ph.D. in physics from Cambridge.

The film proved useful as a scientific tool as well. Since each new layer of the substance reflected light slightly differently, each appeared to reflect a different color. By making a "color gauge," matching the number of layers to the color reflected, Blodgett was able to determine the exact thickness of the film. It is now used to measure very small thicknesses in physics, metallurgy, and chemistry.

Blodgett continued her work with the film, which had been renamed the Langmuir-Blodgett film, until her retirement from General Electric at age sixty-five. She died sixteen year later, in 1979.

TO FIND OUT MORE . . .

- Vare, Ethlie Ann and Ptacek, Greg. *Mothers of Invention: Forgotten Women and Their Unforgettable Ideas.* New York: William Morrow & Co., 1988.

- Yost, Edna. *American Women of Science.* New York: J.B. Lippincott Company, 1955.

Alice Middleton Boring, 1883-1955

A lice Boring had an exciting scientific career that spanned three fields and two countries. Adventurous and energetic, she shaped her work to fit whatever circumstances she happened to find herself in at the time. After eighteen years' work in genetics and cell biology, Boring changed course completely and went to China to work in amphibian and reptile taxonomy. Despite near-impossible working conditions—World War II put her in a Shantung concentration camp—Boring worked for the rest of her life to bridge the gap between Chinese and Western science.

Elizabeth and Edward Boring made their home in Philadelphia and had four children there. Edward was a pharmacist. Alice Boring went to Friends Central School in the city and was accepted at Bryn Mawr upon her graduation in 1900.

At Bryn Mawr she earned a B.A., an M.A., and a Ph.D. over the next ten years, following a conservative course under several excellent professors in cytology and genetics, including Nettie Stevens and Thomas Hunt Morgan. Her doctoral work investigated the behavior of chromosomes in the formation of spermatozoa in insects.

Boring worked as an instructor at Vassar's biology department in 1907 and 1908 and spent some time at the University of Würtzburg in Germany in 1908 and 1909. After Bryn Mawr awarded her a Ph.D. in 1910, she taught for eight years at the University of Maine's zoology department with biologists Gilman Drew and Raymond Pearl. Although she did well in the conventional track of research and teaching, something was missing for her. In 1918, she accepted a position as an assistant professor of biology at a medical college in Peking.

She fell in love with the country. After her two years were up, she returned to the States for a few years, teaching zoology at Wellesley, but returned to China as soon as possible, this time taking a temporary job as a biology instructor at Peking University. She involved herself in China's turbulent politics, speaking out against the West's tendency toward intervention. She immersed herself in the study of China's lizards and amphibians, which were not well understood by Western scientists. Her Chinese students had the benefit of her thorough understanding of their country's fauna and her Western point of view, and she was able to act as a sort of bridge between East and West in her work.

War interrupted her work. The Japanese invasion in 1937 made the atmosphere in Peking University (renamed Yenching University) foreboding. Money was tight, and mail delivery was sporadic. Boring, who felt she had more than most, loaned out most of her money to friends. In 1941, the English and American faculty of the University were placed in a concentration camp in Shantung. In a letter to her family when she was repatriated in 1943, she wrote with remarkable good spirits that "we have been marvelously well" during the ordeal.

After her return, Boring took positions at Columbia University and Mount Holyoke. She brought her American students her deep interest in Chinese herpetology, again acting as a bridge between scientific understanding in the east and the west. In 1946, she was again able to return to Yenching University. Back in the political thick of things, she began to take a cautiously hopeful attitude toward China's Communist party, even in the midst of civil war. It was not the dangerous situation in her adopted country that finally brought her back to the States in 1950, but the illness of her sister.

Boring moved to Cambridge, Massachusetts, and was a part-time professor of zoology at Smith College. She was eighty-one when she died.

> *Boring spent over a year in a concentration camp in Shantung, China.*

TO FIND OUT MORE . . .

- Ogilvie, Marilyn Bailey. *Women in Science*. Cambridge, MA: The MIT Press, 1986.

Sara Elizabeth Branham, 1888–1962

· ·

Like **Hattie Elizabeth Alexander**, Sara Branham conducted extensive and pioneering work on meningitis, a frightening, often fatal infectious disease that attacks the membrane around the brain and spinal cord. Branham was the first to demonstrate that sulfa drugs successfully inhibited the activity of meningococcal bacteria, making Sulfadiazine the best new weapon against meningitis.

Branham's childhood and young adult years were spent near her hometown of Oxford, Georgia. She attended Wesleyan College in nearby Macon, majoring in biology, then taught biology in Atlanta until 1917, when she became an assistant in bacteriology at the University of Colorado. In 1923, she earned a Ph.D. (magna cum laude) from Colorado, and decided to continue studying for a medical degree.

Before she completed her M.D., she was offered a position as a bacteriologist at the Hygienic Laboratories of the United States Public Health Service (now the National Institute of Health, or NIH). She earned her M.D. during a brief leave of absence from the NIH, in 1934. With the exception of this brief leave, Branham would remain at the Institute for thirty years. Most of her work on meningitis was done for the NIH.

At Chicago, Branham had worked with *bacterium enteritidis*, a type of bacteria that causes food poisoning (salmonella). By the time she joined the NIH in 1927, however, meningitis had become a far more serious problem in the United States, with an epidemic that was sweeping from California eastward, and she became involved in the fight against the disease.

The last epidemic had hit the United States more than a decade before, and the antiserum that had been developed to fight that earlier outbreak was not effective against the new strain of bacteria, *Neisseria meningitidis*. Worse, any work with meningococci was extremely labor-intensive, since the cultures needed to be subcultured every other day in order to keep the strain viable.

Branham led several battles against the disease. She traveled to England to bring back strains of dead meningitis bacteria, used to identify live samples sent her at the NIH. She identified several different strains of meningococci. She explored the mechanics of the new epidemic, demonstrating that the type and virulence of the meningococcus was a more important factor in the spread of the disease than the number of infected people in the population. And in 1937, she found that sulfa drugs were effective in treating meningitis. When another epidemic threatened around 1940, it was efficiently squelched by sulfa drugs and newer, more effective antisera.

Branham continued her work at NIH until her retirement in 1958 at age seventy. She continued to contribute significantly, studying the effects of various toxins in mice, chicks and monkeys. She was named Woman of the Year in 1959 by the American Medical Women's Association. She died in 1962.

A pioneering researcher in the field of public health, Branham helped to fight meningitis in the first half of the century.

TO FIND OUT MORE . . .

- O'Hern, Elizabeth Moot. *Profiles of Pioneer Women Scientists*. New York: Acropolis Books, 1985.
- Pittman, M. "Sarah Elizabeth Branham (Matthews): A Biographical Sketch." *ASM News* 42: 420–22.

Emma Lucy Braun, 1889–1971

Ecologist E. Lucy Braun used her knowledge of botany to work for the conservation of natural habitats in and around her home in Cincinnati, Ohio. With her sister, entomologist Annette Braun, she turned the home they shared into a small laboratory with a botanical garden. She was a major contributor to the understanding of North American flora in a more general sense as well: she undertook one of the first studies comparing Ohio plants of the 1900s with plants of the same region from a century before.

Both sisters grew up in Cincinnati. Their mother, Emma Moriah Wright Braun, was an amateur botanist who kept a collection of dried plant specimens for study. Their father, a school principal, joined her in encouraging the two girls in their interest in the outdoors. Emma (she later preferred to be known as E. Lucy) and Annette went on educational trips to the woods to identify plant wildlife.

Braun's formal education was in the public schools and at the University of Cincinnati. She plowed straight through her bachelor's degree (1910), her master's in geology (1912), and her Ph.D. in botany (1924), which she earned just before her twenty-fifth birthday. She stayed at the University to go through the ranks in similarly orderly fashion, rising from assistant in botany in 1914 to associate professor of botany in 1927.

Her publications were extensive and authoritative. She spent much of her life in and around Cincinnati and was a leading authority on Ohio plant life. In the 1920s and 1930s she conducted her pioneering study comparing the current Ohio flora with the flora of one hundred years before. At this time, Braun also began the long period of comprehensive field work that led to the publication of her definitive *Deciduous Forests of Eastern North America* (1950). In 1935 she became the first woman president of the Ohio Academy of Science.

Despite these contributions, Braun was not made a full professor until two years before her retirement from the University of Cincinnati in 1948 at the age of fifty-nine. She was, if anything, more productive after her retirement than before, continuing to conduct field research and to publish major works. In 1951 she established and headed the Ohio Flora Committee under the auspices of the Ohio Academy of Science.

She continued to analyze as well as catalog the flora of her home state. In a 1955 study, "The Phytogeography of Unglaciated Eastern United States and Its Interpretation," she argued that surviving plant populations in the Southern Appalachians gave rise to other forest communities. After glaciers wiped out most plant life, these were the ones from which new life sprang.

Braun was a dedicated conservationist who used her own home as a conservatory for studying rare and odd plants. She and her sister lived in Mount Washington, near Cincinnati. Their house was a laboratory, their garden experimental, and the woods near the house a natural preserve. Braun established a chapter of the Wild Flower Preservation Society in Cincinnati and wrote tireless articles arguing for the conservation of wildlife habitats. She died at home at the age of eighty-one.

Despite an enviable list of contributions in her field, Braun had to wait twenty-one years to earn a full professorship at the University of Cincinnati.

TO FIND OUT MORE ...

- Peskin, Perry K. "A Walk Through Lucy Braun's Prairie." *The Explorer* 20, no. 4 (1978): 15–20.

- Sicherman, Barbara, and Carol Hurd Green, eds. *Notable American Women: The Modern Period. A Biographical Dictionary.* Cambridge, MA: The Belknap Press of Harvard University Press, 1980.

- Stuckey, Ronald L. "E. Lucy Braun (1889–1971), Outstanding Botanist and Conservationist: A Biographical Sketch, with Bibliography." *Mich. Botanist,* 12 (1973): 83–106.

Augusta Fox Bronner, 1881–1966

C linical psychologist Augusta Fox Bronner was a specialist in the psychology of juvenile delinquents. At the age of fifty, she married her former mentor and long-time collaborator, sixty-three-year-old William Healy, and together they established a clinic in Boston to follow up their diagnostic psychiatric work with counseling. The clinic was one of the first of its kind, a model for countless others both in America and abroad.

Bronner's Louisville, Kentucky, childhood was a happy and comfortable one. Her father was a wholesaler who dealt in hats, and her mother was an independent-minded woman who thought her daughter should grow up to pursue a career. Augusta did not learn to do housework; she planned, from the age of six, to become a teacher.

In her first year teaching in 1901, she showed an aptitude for handling difficult students when she tamed a batch of unruly fourth graders. In 1903 she enrolled at Columbia University's Teachers College. As a student, she secured a position as an assistant to educational psychologist Edward L. Thorndike. After her graduation, she spent the five years until her father's death teaching at the girls' school that was her alma mater.

Bronner returned to Teachers College in 1911, once again assisting Edward Thorndike and pushing on for her doctorate in psychology. Her doctoral thesis was a groundbreaking study of delinquent and mentally deficient girls. She found no evidence to show that retarded girls were more likely to behave destructively than normal girls, showing that something less quantifiable determines such behavior. The study, published when Bronner received her Ph.D. in 1914, became a classic, and contributed to the understanding of both delinquent behavior and the behavior of the mentally disabled.

A summer school course at Harvard in 1913 had introduced Bronner to neurologist William Healy. He taught a class on the motivation of juvenile offenders, and she impressed him with her aptitude and dedication. He hired her after her graduation to work as a psychologist at the Chicago Juvenile Psychopathic Institute. The work there was in research, which struggled under the major limitation that no follow-up work was possible for the Institute's young subjects. Bronner found a solution in Boston, where she was able to secure funding from wealthy patrons to found a clinic to provide follow-up care for young offenders. She enlisted Healy to help, and in 1917 they opened the Judge Baker Foundation, later renamed the Judge Baker Children's Center, in Boston.

The Judge Baker Foundation was the focus of the rest of both their professional lives, until they retired together in 1946. Healy and Bronner were married in 1932, after his previous wife died. Their work at the Foundation made them authorities on troubled children and criminal behavior. Bronner lectured at Boston University, Simmons College, and the FBI training school. Despite her considerable knowledge, Bronner seemed content to let her older, better-established husband take the limelight, and she focused on helping her young charges instead of publishing.

Bronner and Healy retired at the ages of sixty-five and seventy-seven. They moved to Clearwater, Florida, where Bronner died twenty years later at the age of eighty-five.

Seventy-six years after its founding, the Judge Baker Children's Center still offers outreach programs to children in the Boston area.

Bronner's groundbreaking study of delinquent and mentally deficient girls became a classic.

TO FIND OUT MORE . . .

- Sicherman, Barbara, and Carol Hurd Green, eds. *Notable American Women: The Modern Period. A Biographical Dictionary.* Cambridge, MA: The Belknap Press of Harvard University Press, 1980.

- Bronner's papers are in the Ethel Sturges Dummer Papers in the Schlesinger Library at Radcliffe College, and at the Judge Baker Guidance Center archives in the Francis A. Countway Library of Medicine, Boston.

Alice Isabel Bever Bryan, 1902–1992

Psychologist Alice Bever Bryan saw reading as a therapeutic tool. Reading, she argued, could help maintain mental equilibrium. Although bibliotherapy had been used after World War I to treat mentally troubled veterans, Bryan's work pioneered its use for healthy people.

Alice Bever was the first of two children born to Caroline and Ewald Bever. She grew up in Kearney, New Jersey, among her extended family; her paternal grandmother lived with the family, and her father's siblings lived nearby with their families. She learned to read and write at home from her doting mother and grandmother, so when she went to public school she started in second grade at age five. She skipped another year in seventh grade, and as a fifteen-year-old senior began teaching as a substitute teacher in the public grammar school.

Bever was encouraged by her teachers to take advantage of the new wartime job openings for women on her graduation in

1918. She decided on a career in publishing and moved to New York, where she attended a secretarial/business program at Columbia University and worked for the American Book Company. New York was exciting for Bever, who was still in her teens. She went out, joined a study group, and took evening classes at Columbia and NYU.

In 1921, Bever began to teach an advertising course through the Y.M.C.A. One of the texts used in the course, *The Psychology of Advertising and Selling*, first attracted her attention to psychology. In 1924, she married Chester Ward Bryan, a mechanical engineer twelve years her senior. Chester Bryan did not want children, so Alice Bryan decided to study to become a psychologist. Through Columbia University, she earned a B.S. in 1929, a master's degree in 1930, and her Ph.D. in 1934, grounding her work with supplemental courses in the anatomy and physiology of the brain in order to be as thoroughly prepared as possible. Her dissertation was written on the correlation between memory and verbal ability in five-year-olds.

While the Bryans had been focused on their separate scientific paths, they had drifted apart. They divorced (amicably) the year Alice Bryan earned her Ph.D. Through several briefly held teaching positions and a grant or two, Bryan published several articles on varied subjects, including one on the differences among women on different career paths. After she married a sculptor and single parent, Frank Marvin Blasingame, in 1936, Bryan was hired as a consulting psychologist and associate in library service at a master's degree program, the School of Library Service at Columbia University. In 1939 she was made assistant professor.

> *Although bibliotherapy had been used after World War I to treat mentally troubled veterans, Bryan's work pioneered its use for healthy people.*

At Columbia, Bryan developed the concept of bibliotherapy, reading as a way to bolster mental health. Bibliotherapy was originally used in veterans' hospitals during and after World War I for the mentally ill. Bryan's bibliotherapy, however, was developed for both well and ill people, as a preventative measure. During World War II, her studies began to be put into practical use in public libraries nationwide. The A.L.A and the A.A.A.P. jointly carried out Bryan's program, designed to bolster civilian morale. Around the same time, Bryan and a group of her peers established the National Council of Women Psychologists.

After her second amicable divorce in 1944, Bryan struggled for a number of years to win academic recognition (and promotion) at Columbia. In 1948, she won a prestigious appointment to conduct a nationwide study of public libraries. She published a book on her findings in 1952, *The Public Librarian*, and was promoted to full professor in 1956. She also conducted a study of doctoral programs that led to the expansion of her own program to include a Ph.D. degree.

Bryan's third marriage, to retired Air Force Colonel George Virgil Fuller, was happy but brief; they were wed in 1956 and he died in 1960. She continued to work at Columbia, in time appointing four of her women students to professorial positions in the program. In 1971, Bryan officially retired at the age of sixty-eight.

TO FIND OUT MORE . . .

- O'Connell, Agnes N., and Nancy Felipe Russo. *Models of Achievement: Reflections of Eminent Women in Psychology.* New York: Columbia University Press, 1983.

Mary Whiton Calkins, 1863–1930

. . . .

One of the true pioneers of psychology, Mary Whiton Calkins began her career as one of the first generation of women to enter the field.

The eldest child of five born to the Reverend Wolcott Calkins and Charlotte Calkins, Mary Calkins was born in Hartford, Connecticut, and spent most of her childhood in Buffalo, New York. Her devotion to her close-knit Protestant family was not unusual for a middle-class American woman of her era, but it was a significant force in her life. In 1881 the family moved to Newton, Massachusetts, where Mary's father had been asked to be the pastor of a Congregational church. In 1882, despite the skepticism with which higher education for women was generally viewed, Calkins left for Smith College.

After Smith, where Calkins studied philosophy and classics, a position as a Greek teacher became available at Wellesley College, only a few miles away from her family's home in Newton. Mary took it gladly and was quickly noticed for her talent as a teacher. Her interest in philosophy made her a candidate for a new position in experimental psychology, provided that she spend a year studying the subject. Calkins accepted the challenge.

Unfortunately, women were not then accepted as students at either Clark University or Harvard University, where Calkins wanted to take classes. She had to circumvent the universities' regulations, writing petitions and working out special arrangements to gain access to the teachings of such luminaries as Josiah Royce, William James, and Edmund C. Sanford. She succeeded in setting up a working laboratory at Wellesley—one of only a handful that existed at the time.

Calkins continued to excel at Harvard with her research on dreams and memory, creating a technique new to psychology. The paired-associate technique, in which subjects are shown a series of numbers paired with colors, proved to be an effective method of enhancing learning. The technique is now standard and widely used. She made short work of all the requirements for the Ph.D. in psychology, and her professors were strongly supportive of her application for the degree. Harvard University, however, simply did not award degrees to women in the 1890s, and Calkins returned to Wellesley without a degree. If Harvard refused to recognize her achievements with a degree, however, Wellesley welcomed her back with enthusiasm, and she began a new phase in her career.

Calkins was the first woman president of the American Psychological Association.

Back at Wellesley, where she would remain for the rest of her nearly forty-year career, Calkins began to develop a new theory of psychology that was at odds with those of the militant behaviorists who dominated her field. By 1900 she had begun to articulate a theory that emphasized the existence of a self independent of other influences. She spent much of her time modifying and defending this pioneering school of thought, which has since become the dominant one. (It has been argued that her rich social and professional life at Wellesley, which functioned as a sort of extended family, influenced her conviction that selves were real and functional in everyday interactions.) On her retirement in 1929, shortly before her death, she was noted as the founder of this school; sadly, however, she is not acknowledged as a forerunner in many recent works on self-psychology.

Calkins' work was celebrated in her day as groundbreaking. Although Harvard had snubbed her, her eminence in her field soon overshadowed this early slight. In 1909 and 1910, Columbia University and Smith University awarded her honorary degrees. As early as 1903 she was ranked twelfth on a list of fifty top psychologists compiled by her peers; two years later she was elected the fourteenth president of the American Psychological Association; and in 1918 she was made the president of the American Philosophical Association. She was the first woman president of either organization.

TO FIND OUT MORE . . .

- Furumoto, L. "Mary Whiton Calkins (1863–1930)." *Psychology of Women Quarterly* 5: 55–68.

- James, E.T. and J.W. *Notable American Women, 1607–1950: A Biographical Dictionary.* Vol. 1. Cambridge, MA: Belknap Press, 1971.

- O'Connell, Agnes N., and Nancy Felipe Russo, eds. *Women in Psychology: A Bio-Bibliographic Sourcebook.* New York: Greenwood Press, 1990.

Annie Jump Cannon, 1863-1941

A nnie Jump Cannon's work in astronomy made her an eminent figure in her field. She was one of the first woman astronomers taken seriously enough to be given a full-fledged position at Harvard as the William Cranch Bond Astronomer. She simplified the existing system of classification and produced an immense body of work that catalogued the stars.

Annie Cannon was the oldest of three children born to Mary and Wilson Cannon. Wilson Cannon was a Delaware state senator who had cast Delaware's deciding vote against secession from the Union, siding the state with the North. Mary Wilson was an amateur astronomer who made a sort of home observatory in the family attic. Annie and her mother spent many nights watching the skies together.

When Annie Cannon went to Wellesley in 1880, the college was only five years old. She studied astronomy under Sarah Whiting until 1884, then spent nearly a decade at home in Dover, where she lived the life of a genteel young woman in polite society. When her mother died in 1893, she returned to Wellesley for postgraduate study with Whiting, then attended Radcliffe as a special student until 1897. She earned her master's degree from Wellesley in 1907.

The director of the Harvard Observatory, Edward Pickering, hired Cannon in 1896 as an assistant on his team. Harvard was to be her professional home for the rest of her life. She was one of several prominent women astronomers who came to Harvard in the early 1900s; her co-workers under Pickering included **Antonia Maury** and Wilhemina Fleming. A patient and skilled observer, Cannon rose steadily at Harvard, succeeding Wilhemina Fleming as curator of the University's collection of astronomical photographs in 1911.

In 1918, Cannon undertook a massive project, *The Henry Draper Catalogue*, with Edward Pickering. When Pickering died in

1919, she continued with the project, which was not completed until after her own death over two decades later. The combined *Henry Draper Catalogue* and *Henry Draper Extension* classified 350,000 different stars. Her other nine catalogues and many articles, including her influential work on variable stars, represented a broad and active career.

Cannon's contributions were recognized by her peers with many honors and appointments. In 1938, her appointment as William Cranch Bond Astronomer at Harvard made her one of the first women appointed to any position at the university. She was made an honorary member of the Royal Astronomical Society in 1914. Her prizes include the National Academy of Sciences' Draper Medal, in 1931, and the Ellen Richards Prize of the Society to Aid Scientific Research by Women, in 1932. She also had a prize for women astronomers named after her and was awarded honorary degrees by Oxford and the University of Groningen.

Annie Cannon worked at Harvard until her death in 1941. She was seventy-eight.

> *Cannon simplified the existing system of classifying stars and produced an immense body of work cataloging them.*

TO FIND OUT MORE . . .

- *Dictionary of Scientific Biography,* Vol. III, pp. 49–50. New York: Charles Scribner's Sons, 1971.

- Ogilvie, Marilyn Bailey. *Women in Science.* Cambridge, MA: The MIT Press, 1986.

Emma Perry Carr, 1880–1972

. . . .

As the head of Mount Holyoke College's chemistry department for over thirty years, Emma Perry Carr led its pioneering research in both organic and physical chemistry. Carr kept her department on the cutting edge by studying abroad on her own time and by using new, difficult techniques like absorption spectroscopy. Her research group made significant strides toward elucidating the complex problems it investigated. Despite her intense involvement with research, Carr's special talent lay in balancing her ambitious investigative work with her considerable contributions to campus life as a teacher, mentor, and administrator.

Emma Perry Carr was the third of five children born to Edmund Cone and Mary Jack Carr. Less then a year after her birth in Holmesville, Ohio, the family moved to Coshocton, Ohio, where Edmund practiced medicine and Mary was active in the Methodist church. Emma Carr grew up in Coshocton, attended the local high schools, and entered nearby Ohio State University in 1898.

After a year at Ohio, she transferred to Mount Holyoke College, where she studied for two years and worked as an assistant in chemistry for three. She finished her B.S. at the University of Chicago in 1905, and after another three years at Mount Holyoke, this time as an instructor, returned to Chicago to earn her Ph.D. in chemistry. After she was awarded her doctorate in 1910, she returned to Mount Holyoke for good.

In 1913 Carr was promoted from associate professor of chemistry to full professor and head of the department. Despite the fact that Mount Holyoke was not a large, well-endowed research university, Carr set about that very year making the chemistry department an important research facility.

With her colleague, organic chemist Dorothy Hahn, Carr led groups of students in a series of group research projects. The most important of these spanned most of the time she spent there and involved the synthesis and analysis by absorption spectroscopy of complex organic compounds. Ultraviolet absorption spectroscopy had not then been much explored in the United States, so Carr traveled to Ireland and Germany to learn all she could about the new technique.

In the late 1920s the group shifted focus slightly and began to analyze simple unsaturated hydrocarbons. In the process of these investigations, they were able to contribute significantly to the understanding of the carbon-carbon double bond, a very important link in chemistry. Their work began to attract attention, and in the 1930s Carr was awarded prestigious grants from the Rockefeller Foundation and the National Research Council. She was recognized with honorary degrees and the Garvan Medal for distinguished service in chemistry by an American woman.

Meanwhile, she led the group to publish thirty-six papers in thirty-three years. She inspired her students to produce work of high quality, and they went on to careers in science more often than graduates of any other women's institution. Carr stepped

> *Carr kept her pioneering department on the cutting edge by studying abroad and by using new techniques.*

down in 1946, but remained involved with campus life until she moved to a rest home in Evanstown, Illinois, in 1964, at the age of eighty-four. She died there eight years later.

TO FIND OUT MORE . . .

- *The National Cyclopedia of American Biography* F, p. 364. New York: J.T. White.

  - Sicherman, Barbara, and Carol Hurd Green, eds. *Notable American Women: The Modern Period. A Biographical Dictionary.* Cambridge, MA: The Belknap Press of Harvard University Press, 1980.

  - Carr's papers are in the archives of the chemistry department and in the Williston Memorial Library at Mount Holyoke College.

Rachel Carson, 1907–1964

Conservationist Rachel Carson once said, "If there is poetry in my book about the sea, it is not because I deliberately put it there, but because no one could write truthfully about the sea and leave out poetry." Certainly her twin loves, biology and writing, are inseparable in the work for which she is best known, *Silent Spring*. This slim volume, an urgent warning about the poisons pumped into our water, soil, and atmosphere by industry and agriculture, marked the birth of the environmental movement.

Carson, who first published a piece in a magazine at age ten, was an introverted young student, excelling in her public high school and attending Pennsylvania College for Women on a scholarship. She started out in the English department, but in her junior year became so entranced with a required biology class that she switched majors. The inspirational professor who taught the course, Mary Scott Skinker, helped her to win a scholarship in 1929 at Johns Hopkins University, where she studied genetics and zoology.

Hopkins provided a solid scientific background for the enthusiastic young student, but her imagination was truly fired in her summers at the Woods Hole Marine Biological Laboratory on Cape Cod. She had only read about the ocean before Woods Hole, but she fell in love with it at once. Carson earned an A.M. in zoology in 1932. In 1935 she found herself in need of a job when her sister died, leaving two children to the care of Rachel and her mother. She became a junior aquatic biologist at the United States Bureau of Fisheries in Washington, D.C.

At the Bureau, Carson resumed her writing, publishing articles in the Baltimore *Sunday Sun*. A 1937 article in the Atlantic Monthly, "Undersea," attracted the attention of an editor at Simon and Schuster. She turned the article into her first book, *Under the Sea-Wind*, which sold poorly when it was published immediately before Pearl Harbor. It was well reviewed, however, and made the best-seller lists when it was reissued a decade later.

Carson spent the years during and after the war running the publications program for the Fish and Wildlife Service. As biologist and chief editor there, she had little time for her writing, and her commitment to her family kept her from considering writing as a career. But she used her spare time to write *The Sea Around Us*, which made her famous when it was published in 1951. It was a best seller for a year and a half, won the National Book Award, and was serialized in the *New Yorker*. Carson's obvious mastery of her subject prompted one reviewer (of questionable intelligence, considering his comment and the fact her full name was on the cover) to write, "I assume from the author's knowledge that he must be a man."

> *Carson's Silent Spring probably ranks as one of the most important books of the century.*

The success of the book and a Guggenheim Fellowship made it possible for Carson to devote herself full-time to writing. She moved to Sheepscott Bay in Maine, where she built a home overlooking the water. She published *The Edge of the Sea* in 1955, which helped confirm her position as a writer who brought the natural world to life for her audience. In 1957 she adopted her five-year-old grandnephew when one of her two nieces died.

A year later she began *Silent Spring*. It was a labor of love, considering her failing health (she was eventually confined to a wheelchair) and the knowledge that her message would not be popular with the powerful agricultural chemical industry, her primary target. But the book prompted governmental measures to curb the use of DDT and other wildlife-killing chemicals; President Kennedy's special panel of the Science Advisory Committee moved to examine the impact of pesticides on the environment.

Carson died only two years after completing *Silent Spring*. Since her death, environmental awareness has increased dramatically, due in no small part to Carson's work. To quote one editorial, "A few thousand words from her, and the world took a different direction."

TO FIND OUT MORE . . .

- Bonta, Margaret Meyers. *Women in the Field: America's Pioneering Naturalists.* College Station, TX: Texas A&M University Press, 1991.

- Brooks, Paul. *The House of Life: Rachel Carson at Work.* New York: Houghton Mifflin, 1972.

- Carson, Rachel. *Silent Spring.* New York: Fawcett Press, 1962.

- Sicherman, Barbara, and Carol Hurd Green, eds. *Notable American Women: The Modern Period. A Biographical Dictionary.* Cambridge, MA: The Belknap Press of Harvard University Press, 1980.

- Sterling, Philip. *Sea and Earth: The Life of Rachel Carson.* New York: Crowell, 1970.

Mary Agnes Meara Chase, 1869–1963

. . . .

The botanist Agnes Chase had no formal training, no college or graduate degree and no childhood background in science. Through sheer love of her subject she was able to turn a pleasant hobby into a distinguished career and contribute significantly to the study of grasses.

The second youngest of six children born to a railroad engineer from Tipperary, Ireland, Mary Agnes Meara was born in Iroquois County, Illinois. Martin J. Meara died when Mary Agnes was only two, and Mary Brannick Meara moved her brood to Chicago. Agnes was helping her mother pay the bills as soon as she was out of grammar school.

As a teenager she took a job at the *School Herald* setting type and reading proof. The editor there, thirty-four-year-old William Ingraham Chase, fell in love with her; they were married in 1888. Agnes was eighteen years old. Less than a year later, William Chase died and left her saddled with his debts. She tightened her belt, taking another proofreading job and working in Chase's brother's general store in Wady Petra, Illinois. Agnes saved money by living on a diet of beans and oatmeal. According to her nephew, she first developed an interest in botany in the store, where she pored over a field guide to wildflowers with him.

Throughout the 1890s Agnes collected the flora of northern Illinois, first as a hobby, later as an increasingly serious occupation. A bryologist friend, Rev. Ellsworth Hill, enlisted her as an illustrator, which led to her work on two Field Museum of Natural History publications. He also introduced her to the compound microscope and encouraged her to apply for a position as an illustrator for the USDA's Bureau of Plant Industry. She got the job—and a $720-per-year salary—and moved to Washington, D.C., in 1903.

At the Bureau, she met the specialist in grasses Albert Spear Hitchcock and began a collaboration that lasted over thirty years. She moved up through the ranks, becoming in succession an assistant in systematic agrostology (the study of grasses), an assistant botanist, and an associate botanist. She took Hitchcock's place as senior botanist and principal scientist in charge of systematic agrostology when he stepped down in 1936.

In her work at the Bureau, Chase made great contributions to agrostology. Her work had important practical applications in agriculture, where the information she painstakingly collected could be applied to develop more robust and nutritious crops. Her many collecting trips to Brazil, Mexico, Puerto Rico, and parts of the U.S. yielded over 4,500 distinct specimens. She donated most of her material to the Smithsonian and the National Herbarium.

Chase was as passionate about her political causes as she was about her work. A dedicated suffragist, she marched for the women's vote during World War I. Despite her unimposing appearance (she was under five feet tall and weighed about ninety-three pounds), she was jailed and then force-fed when she went on a hunger strike. She also supported Prohibition and donated gener-

> *Chase's work helped in the development of more robust and nutritious crops.*

ously to the Fellowship of Reconciliation, the NAACP, the National Women's Party, and the Women's International League for Peace and Freedom.

Physically active into her nineties, Chase continued to work for the National Herbarium long after her 1936 retirement. She continued to take field trips, including one to Venezuela in her seventies. She cared for an aging sister for nearly twenty years, although she was herself in her seventies and eighties, and finally moved in with her longtime friend Florence Van Eseltine at age eighty-four. She died ten years later at a nursing home in Bethesda, Maryland.

TO FIND OUT MORE . . .

- Ogilve, Marilyn Bailey. *Women in Science.* Cambridge, MA: The MIT Press, 1986.

- Sicherman, Barbara, and Carol Hurd Green, eds. *Notable American Women: The Modern Period. A Biographical Dictionary.* Cambridge, MA: The Belknap Press of Harvard University Press, 1980.

- Chase's papers are at the Hunt Institute for Botanical Documentation at Carnegie–Mellon University.

May Edward Chinn, 1896–1980

When May Chinn began practicing medicine in New York City in the late twenties, African-American physicians could not be officially affiliated with New York hospitals. Despite this considerable handicap, she conducted research in cancer for nearly fifty years. Twelve of those years were spent working with George Papanicolaou, whose "pap smear" test makes possible early detection of cervical cancer. Meanwhile, she maintained a busy private practice in Harlem.

May Chinn was the only child of Lula Ann Evans Chinn, an African-American/Native American, and William Lafayette Chinn, a former slave. The couple had moved to Great Barrington, Massachusetts, from Virginia. Lula Ann Chinn, who worked as a domestic servant, backed her daughter when she wanted to go back to school. Because May had not finished high school, she had to take a series of tests to qualify for college admissions. She passed the examinations

and moved to New York City to enroll at Teachers' College at Columbia University, where she earned her bachelor's degree in 1921.

Chinn enrolled at The University of Bellevue Medical Center (later the University Medical College at New York University) to pursue her medical degree. She earned the degree at age thirty, in 1926. She spent a year practicing medicine in Harlem, treating all comers, before she decided to do research in cancer. She spent the five years from 1928 until 1933 working with Papanicolaou at Columbia. The university awarded her an M.S. in public health in 1933.

From 1930 to 1977, Chinn maintained both her private practice in Harlem and her cancer research. Although she did not specialize, she enjoyed treating women and children and always worked in at least one children's clinic. She often waived or reduced fees for patients who were unable to pay in full. Although she ran her own practice as much as a public service as a business, she also found time to be involved with other public service organizations, working in a range of clinics. From 1948 to 1955, she worked once more with Papanicolaou at Cornell University, studying exfoliative cytology.

In 1975 Chinn co-founded the Susan Smith McKinney Steward, M.D. Society, which two years later selected her as an honoree. The Society was organized to promote African-American women in medicine. Chinn was also recognized by both her alma maters, Columbia and New York University, with honorary degrees.

> *The daughter of a former slave, Chinn conducted important cancer research for half a century.*

Chinn officially retired in 1977, at age eighty-one. She was vigorously active right up to her death, working for the American Cancer Society and as a consultant for the Phelps-Stokes Fund, which paid for African and other foreign students to study in America. She died at age eighty-four.

TO FIND OUT MORE . . .

- Smith, Jessie Carey. *Notable Black American Women.* Detroit, MI: Gale Research Inc., 1992.

- *Who's Who of Americans with World Notables.* Chicago: Marquis, 1970-71.

- Transcripts of Chinn's interviews with the Black Women Oral History Project are at the Schlesinger Library at Radcliffe College.

Edith Clarke, 1883–1959

Edith Clarke, "Member No. 1" of the Society of Women Engineers, has been called the foremost woman engineer in history. She is remembered for her many "firsts" as a woman in her field: She was the first woman elected to the Society of Electrical Engineers, the first woman to recieve a master's degree in electrical engineering from MIT, and the first woman to teach electrical engineering in an American university. But her contributions to her field were prodigious and ought not to be overlooked.

Edith Clarke was born on Feb. 10, 1883, in Howard County, Maryland. Her father, a lawyer and gentleman farmer, died when Edith was only seven years old; her mother ran the farm until her death five years later, which left Edith and her siblings orphaned. An uncle was appointed guardian, and the oldest daughter, Mary, raised the younger children. Edith had the freedom to use her share of the inheritance as she chose, and although some of her relatives chastised her for it, she spent the money on college tuition.

At Vassar, Clarke studied math and physics. She wanted to study engineering, but that subject was not offered to young women at Vassar in the early 1900s. After three years spent teaching math and physics, Clarke became seriously ill. Later, she told a reporter, "Thinking I was going to die, I just decided to do what I really wanted to do—study engineering." She trained at the School of Engineering at the University of Wisconsin for a year, worked for the American Telephone & Telegraph Company for another seven, and finally was accepted at MIT to study electrical engineering.

While at MIT, she became interested in symmetrical components, a complicated mathematical technique for quick computing. Although she didn't invent the concept—that credit went to Charles Fortescue—she tinkered with the technique, developing a convenient version that made it workable. In pre-computerization days, equations were worked out by hand. The new components, called "Clarke components," streamlined many complex equations.

Despite her accomplishments as a mathematician and a practical engineer, she was unable upon graduation from MIT to find a position better than her old job at AT&T, where she supervised a pool of "girls" in the computing pool. She moved to Constantinople for a year to teach engineering at the Woman's College in Turkey. On her return, General Electric hired her—at last—as an electrical engineer, analyzing problems of power transmission submitted by power companies throughout the nation. Her work for them spanned twenty-three years, until Clarke was sixty-two. In those years, she placed circut theory on firm mathematical ground. She also published what became the major textbook of her field, *Circut Analysis of AC Power Systems, Symmetrical and Related Components* (1943).

After she left GE, Clarke was made a professor at the University of Texas, Austin. She spent the last nine years of her career there, teaching, publishing, and accepting honors from the American Institute of Electrical Engineers and the Society of Women Engineers.

> *Although Vassar wouldn't offer engineering courses to the young women of the early 1900s, Clarke resolved to study it anyway after she graduated.*

TO FIND OUT MORE . . .

- Farnes, Kass-Simon and Patricia. *Women of Science: Righting the Record.* Bloomington, IL: Indiana University Press, 1990.

- Goff, Alice C. *Women Can Be Engineers.* Youngstown, OH: n.p., 1946.

- Read, Phyllis J., and Bernard L. Witlieb. *The Book of Women's Firsts.* New York: Random House, 1992.

Anna Botsford Comstock, 1854–1930

Naturalist Anna Comstock made lasting contributions to the nature study movement that began around the turn of the century. Alarmed by the exodus of New York farmers from their farms to the cities in search of more lucrative jobs, the state legislature instituted programs designed to make agricultural work more appealing. Among them was Anna Comstock's committee, which taught nature study to farm children. She began to write pamphlets for the committee, and went on to become the author of many popular, gently instructive books like *Ways of the Six-Footed* (1903).

Anna Botsford, an only child, spent her childhood days roaming her Quaker parents' New York State farm. She first fell in love with nature there, following her mother's lead in appreciating the beauty in the world around her. After two years at a Methodist school in Randolph, New York, she taught for a year in her hometown. From 1874 until 1877, Botsford studied lan-

guages and literature at Cornell. She met her husband in an entomology class (he was the professor). They were married at her home in 1878.

Over the next two decades, Anna Comstock devoted her energies to supporting her husband's career. She was his lab assistant and skilled illustrator for many years, and in 1888 her wood carvings for his publications made her one of the first four women to be elected to Sigma Xi, the national science honor society. The couple moved about as John Comstock lectured and conducted research in Washington, D.C., California, and Germany, but eventually settled at Cornell, where Anna Comstock finished her bachelor's degree in natural history in 1885.

Anna Comstock's work with the Committee for the Promotion of Agriculture from 1895 until 1897 helped her win a position at Cornell, which was affiliated with the nature study project. In 1899 she became the first woman to reach professorial status at Cornell when she was hired as an assistant professor of nature study. The board of trustees opposed the existence of a female assistant professor at the university, so her title was dropped to lecturer the next year. She regained her rank in 1913 and was made a full professor in 1920.

As a leading figure in nature study over the next three decades until her death, it has been said that Comstock "inspired probably more men and women to pioneer in a new field then any other person." In addition to her many books, which included the immensely popular 1911 *Handbook of Nature-Study* (in its twenty-fourth edition in 1939), she was a dedicated contributor to nature science organizations and the editor of the *Nature-Study Review*. She seldom missed an important meeting of the American Nature Study Society, and also served as the associate director of the American Nature Association.

Anna Comstock was well loved by her students and her wide readership. In a 1923 poll taken by the League of Women Voters, she was named one of America's twelve greatest living women. She remained active in her many organizations until her death at seventy-five.

> *Named the first woman professor in Cornell's history, Comstock's title was reduced to lecturer after protests from the board of trustees.*

TO FIND OUT MORE . . .

- Ogilvie, Marilyn Bailey. *Women in Science.* Cambridge, MA: The MIT Press, 1986.

- Sicherman, Barbara, and Carol Hurd Green, eds. *Notable American Women: The Modern Period. A Biographical Dictionary.* Cambridge, MA: The Belknap Press of Harvard University Press, 1980.

- Comstock's papers are at the Museum of Comparative Zoology at Harvard University.

Gerty Theresa Radnitz Cori, 1896–1957

In 1947, Gerty Cori and her husband Carl won the Nobel Prize in medicine and physiology as a pair. It was the culmination of almost thirty years of cooperative work; they had first collaborated on research in medical school. In a radio interview, Cori once said: "The love for and dedication to one's work seem to me to be the basis for happiness." The Coris were able to keep that dedication at the center of both their personal and professional lives.

Gerty Cori was born in Prague, the eldest of three girls born to Martha and Otto Radnitz. She was tutored at home and went to a private finishing school until sixteen, when she abruptly decided that she wanted to go to medical school. She attacked the remaining requirements, which included eight years of Latin and five of mathematics, chemistry, and physics. It took her a year to complete them and pass the entrance exam for a six-year medical school program at Carl Ferdinand University.

In school, Gerty met Carl. They decided to wait until they had earned their degrees to marry, but began to collaborate as students. They conducted a study of the immune bodies of blood together and published their findings in a scientific journal in 1920. Later that same year, they graduated and were married.

Although their working relationship was not only equal but fruitful for both researchers, Gerty's gender kept her work from being taken as seriously as Carl's. In 1922, Carl was offered a post as a biochemist at the New York Institute for the Study of Malignant Diseases in Buffalo. Gerty Cori followed a few months later, but she was only able to secure a position as an assistant biochemist there. The director once threatened to fire Gerty if she continued her work with her husband, which the couple pursued in their own spare time. Later, when Carl was considering taking a job at another university, Gerty was told that it was unAmerican for a man to work with his wife and that she was holding her husband back professionally.

The Coris, who became naturalized U.S. citizens in 1928, moved to St. Louis in 1931 to conduct research on normal carbohydrate metabolism (the Buffalo lab focused on cancer). Carl was made the chairman of the Washington University School of Medicine's department of pharmacology, but Gerty had only a research position (and a tiny salary) in the same department. She only became a full professor in 1947, when she was awarded the Nobel Prize.

Together the Coris picked apart the chemical processes of carbohydrate breakdown within a living being. Working with tissue preparations, they found that a substance called the "Cori ester," glucose-1-phosphate, was formed when the enzyme phosphorylase broke down glycogen. They were able to synthesize glycogen in a test tube for the first time in 1939. Their work made it possible for Gerty to clarify the workings of childhood glycogen storage diseases, showing that a hereditary disease could stem from a defect in an enzyme.

> *Although she kept it a secret until after the ceremony awarding her and her husband the Nobel Prize in medicine, Gerty Cori knew that she had myelosclerosis, an incurable bone marrow disease.*

Soon before the award presentation for their Nobel Prize, Gerty and Carl Cori learned that Gerty had myelosclerosis, an incurable bone marrow disease. They told no one until after the ceremony, and Gerty continued to work despite the increasing debility her disease caused. She finally died of kidney failure brought on by myelosclerosis in 1957. The Coris' only child, Carl, born in 1936, grew up to become a research chemist.

TO FIND OUT MORE . . .

- Opfell, Olga S. *The Lady Laureates: Women Who Have Won the Nobel Prize.* Metutchen, NJ: The Scarecrow Press, 1986.

- Sichelman, Barbara, and Carol Hurd Green, eds. *Notable American Women: The Modern Period. A Biographical Dictionary.* Cambridge, MA: The Belknap Press of Harvard University Press, 1980.

- Yost, Edna. *Women of Modern Science.* New York: Dodd, Mead, 1964.

Gladys Rowena Henry Dick, 1881–1963

B efore the introduction of antibiotics during World War II, scarlet fever was a major public health hazard, killing about a quarter of its mostly pre-adolescent victims. Those who survived were often left crippled by the rackingly high fevers—Helen Keller lost her sight and hearing to the disease as a toddler. The microbiologist and physician Gladys Dick, working with her physician husband George Francis Dick, found the bacteria that causes the disease. Working systematically and rapidly, they developed methods of diagnosis, prevention, and treatment of the disease.

Gladys Rowena Henry earned her high school and college degrees in Nebraska. Even so, it took three years, during which she taught high school biology, to convince her mother to let her go to medical school.

She set out for Baltimore to study at Johns Hopkins in 1903. Johns Hopkins did not then provide housing for its female students, so with typical aplomb Henry organized her female peers to buy a house as a group. She earned her M.D. in four years and spent a year doing postgraduate work in Berlin, then a few more doing further study at Hopkins. Focusing on experimental cardiac surgery and blood chemistry, she was able to work with top researchers. In 1911 she moved to Chicago, where her mother had settled, and started the work for which she is best known.

At the University of Chicago she met and married fellow physician George Dick. They had been working together for some time on the etiology of scarlet fever when they wed. After a long honeymoon in Egypt and the Balkans, they returned to Chicago to collaborate on further scarlet fever research at the University's John R. McCormick Memorial Institute for Infectious Diseases, founded in memory of a child who died of scarlet fever and devoted to eradicating the disease.

The Dicks were methodical researchers

who worked for nearly ten years eliminating the technical difficulties of positively identifying the bacteria that caused the disease. In 1923 they announced their findings: Hemolytic streptococci, previously thought to be secondary invaders, was the cause of scarlet fever. In less than a year they developed a skin test based on their finding that the streptococci release a toxin that produces the red rash typical of scarlet fever. The test, called "the Dick test," was immediately usable world-wide, and the team began developing an antiserum.

Gladys Dick, working with her physician husband George Francis Dick, found the bacteria that causes scarlet fever.

Their discoveries made them scientific celebrities. They were jointly considered for the 1925 Nobel Prize in medicine, but none was given that year. Soon, however, their fame changed to a sort of notoriety when they patented their methods of producing both the toxin and an antitoxin, and in so doing started a controversy. The scarlet fever problem had been pursued by others for some time, and while the Dicks were the first to succeed, others were on the same track. Opponents argued that the patents would block further research and biological standardization. Gladys Dick took Lederle Laboratories to court in the late 1920s, claiming patent infringement. To critics accusing them of commercial greed, the Dicks replied that they had not profited financially from their patents and that they sought only to control the quality of others' use of their methods. The Dicks won in court, but the question became a moot one in the 1940s with the development of antibiotics.

At forty-nine Gladys adopted two adored children, Roger Henry and Rowena Henry Dick. Gladys had founded and been active in the Cradle Society, perhaps the first American adoption agency, for over a decade. She split her time between the Cradle Society and polio research, increasingly interested in child welfare in her later years. In 1953 she retired with her husband to Palo Alto, where she fought her draining cerebral arteriosclerosis for ten years. She died in 1963.

TO FIND OUT MORE...

- Obituary. *The Chicago Tribune*, August 23, 1963.

- Sicherman, Barbara, and Carol Hurd Green, eds. *Notable American Women: The Modern Period. A Biographical Dictionary.* Cambridge, MA: The Belknap Press of Harvard University Press, 1980.

- Siegel, Patricia Joan, and Kay Thomas Finley. *Women in the Scientific Search: An American Bio-Bibliography, 1724–1979.* London: The Scarecrow Press, 1985.

Caroline Dorman, 1888-1971

"**A**ll I ask of life is to stay in the woods, fooling with plants and birds," wrote botanist and conservationist Carrie Dormon. She managed to spend most of her life doing just that in her home state, Louisiana.

Carrie Dormon was born at her parents' summer home, Briarwood, in the hills of northwestern Louisiana. Dormon spent a joyful childhood in the outdoors with her brothers and father. She was an asset to her older brothers on their egg-collecting trips because she was so small and light that she could climb out onto the thinnest branches to pluck wild birds' eggs from the nests. Even as a child, however, she had a conservationist's care for nature, and never stole more than one egg from a nest.

At home in Arcadia, Louisiana, she was an intellectually precocious child who began writing at the age of three. At sixteen she was sent to Judson College in Marion, Alabama, for "finishing." She never considered herself tamed by the school, however, and in fact brought a little of the wild to it by teaching her classmates bird calls. She majored in literature and art and, at nineteen, began to teach after her graduation in 1907.

Three tragedies followed in rapid succession: the 1907 death of her mother, her father's death in 1909, and a fire that consumed the family home in Arcadia three months afterward. Dormon became even closer to her sister Virginia, who was twelve years her senior and a mother figure. The sisters moved permanently to the old family summer home, Briarwood, in 1918.

Dormon felt confined by teaching. She disliked spending all of her time indoors and found the role a limiting one. In 1919, she felt that it literally made her sick and asked the school superintendent to find a way to let her work outdoors. The previous year, her enthusiasm for virgin pine forests at a conservation forum led to her appointment as state chairman of conservation for the Louisiana Federation of Women's Clubs. She was transferred to a school in the middle of longleaf virgin pine forests in the hilly Kisatchie area in Natchitoches Parish.

A long fight with red tape to save a portion of this forest was lost when the company that owned the land decided to raze the forest. But her fight launched a career in forestry, which had been what she had wanted to pursue in the first place. Her work with the Louisiana Department of Conservation in 1921–1923 and 1927–1929 was fraught with bureaucratic obstacles, however, and she withdrew permanently to Briarwood after 1930. That same year, she was one of the first three women to be elected to associate membership in the Society of American Foresters.

Dormon found her life's work in Louisiana's rich bounty of uncatalogued irises. With their fantastic variations in color, size, and sinuous form, they were a wonderful subject for an enthusiast like Dormon. She painted, photographed, and collected many new species, corresponding with botanists about her findings. She often took other botanists on collecting trips in Louisiana. Dormon also began breeding irises with Virginia at Briarwood, beginning to sell them in the 1940s.

Dormon wrote most of her books after the late 1950s, when old age kept her indoors more than she might have liked. She wrote wonderfully extensive guides designed for amateurs like herself, written in plain prose. **Rachel Carson**'s *Silent Spring* put new fire in her conservationist efforts at the age of seventy-eight. She wrote her last article on the destruction wrought by the pesticides DDT and heptachlor, both of which are targeted in Carson's book.

In a fitting tribute to this dedicated Louisana botanist, Louisiana State University awarded her an honorary doctorate when she was seventy-seven. After her death, Briarwood was preserved as a botanical sanctuary through the Caroline Dormon Foundation, set up by friends.

> *Champion of Louisiana forests, Dormon wrote guidebooks that opened the wilderness to others.*

TO FIND OUT MORE . . .

- Bonta, Margaret Meyers. *Women in the Field: America's Pioneering Naturalists.* College Station, TX: Texas A&M University Press. 1991.

- Moore, Diane M. *The Adventurous Will: Profiles of Memorable Louisiana Women.* Lafayette, LA: Arcadiana Press, 1984.

- Snell, David. "The Green World of Carrie Dormon." *Smithsonian* 2 (1972): 28.

June Etta Downey, 1875–1932

One of a handful of eminent women psychologists in the early part of the twentieth century, June Etta Downey was one of the first two to be recognized by election to the exclusive Society of Experimental Psychologists in 1929. (In 1947, the organization once again reflected its founder's original vision of "an experimental club with no women.") She was a well-rounded and thoroughly accomplished scientist who published prolifically and was adored by her students; she was also a meticulous researcher whose name was starred in the 1927 edition of *American Men of Science.*

Downey came from a family with a strong tradition of leadership. Her mother was a community organizer in June's Laramie, Wyoming, hometown. Her father, who had been a colonel for the Union Army in the Civil War, served Wyoming as a territorial delegate to Congress. His work in the Wyoming legislature made him instrumental in the founding of the University of Wyoming, which appointed him a member of the board of trustees. Her younger brother Sheridan grew up to be a United States senator for California.

No slouch herself, June Downey majored in classics at the University of Wisconsin and cultivated an interest in experimental science. After graduating in 1895, she enrolled at the University of Chicago, where she received a master's degree in psychology and philosophy in 1898. Later that same year, she returned to Wyoming, where she would spend the rest of her career as an instructor in English.

Downey's interests moved slowly from English to philosophy and, beginning in 1901, psychology. She was made a full professor of English in 1905. She took time off to complete her Ph.D. at Chicago in 1906 and 1907, writing a dissertation on handwriting and personality that was published by the *Psychological Review.* When she was awarded the degree with honors in 1908, she became the first woman head of a state university psychology department.

By 1915 Downey had focused exclusively on psychology. She became an expert in the study of handwriting and handedness (as in left- and right-) and the influence personality has on both voluntary and involuntary movement. She developed a pioneering personality test, which did not endure but nevertheless broke new ground. These were slippery and subjective areas, but Downey's experiments were impeccable in their scientific precision.

At Wisconsin Downey fought spotty health and handled a hefty load of research, writing, and teaching. Despite her busy schedule, she made herself available to her students, acting as a mentor and counselor to many. Her publications were not only scholarly; she retained her love of literature and herself wrote short stories, plays, poems, and nonscientific articles.

Downey's honors included election to the council of the American Psychological Association, on which she served from 1923 to 1925. In 1929, she and **Margaret Floy Washburn** were the first women elected to the Society of Experimental Psychologists. She worked up until her final illness, which struck when she was visiting New York City for the 1932 Third International Congress of Eugenics. She died two months later in her sister's New Jersey home.

> *Downey's pioneering personality test broke new ground.*

TO FIND OUT MORE ...

- Ogilvie, Marilyn Bailey. *Women in Science.* Cambridge, MA: The MIT Press, 1986.

- Scarborough, Elizabeth, and Laurel Furumoto. *Untold Lives: The First Generation of American Women Psychologists.* New York: Columbia University Press, 1987.

- Sicherman, Barbara, and Carol Hurd Green, eds. *Notable American Women: The Modern Period. A Biographical Dictionary.* Cambridge, MA: The Belknap Press of Harvard University Press, 1980.

Cornelia (Cora) Mitchell Downs, 1892-1987

Bacteriologist Cora Downs was a leading expert on tularemia, or "rabbit fever." During the Depression, families strapped for money often hunted for food. In Kansas, where Downs lived for much of her career, the thriving rabbit population often fed the hungry human population. The problem was that the rabbit dinners infected people with the rodent-carried disease, causing an array of exhausting symptoms: recurrent fevers, aches, lesions that wouldn't heal, and swollen lymph nodes.

Downs had a quiet Kansas childhood. She was born in Wyandotte, Kansas, and went to local high schools. She pursued her education at the University of Kansas slowly but methodically, earning her bachelor's degree in bacteriology at age twenty-three, a master's degree at twenty-eight, and her Ph.D. at thirty-two, in 1924. (A plan to move to the University of Chicago to complete her Ph.D. was abandoned when her mother became ill.)

Downs had always been interested in infectious diseases. Her graduate work on streptococci and typhoid fever set the stage for her work on tularemia. Practical considerations played a part as well; research money was hard to come by, and research on tularemia was relatively inexpensive. Downs published her first paper on the disease in 1930.

The research conducted by Downs at Kansas over the next thirteen years focused on developing a vaccine for *Pasteurella tularensis*. She was able to culture the bacteria from a rabbit hunter with a lesion on his finger. She found compounds that killed or impaired the tularemia bacteria, and tested vaccines of dead bacteria on white rats. These vaccines were ineffective, so Downs began looking for a live strain that was weak enough to be overcome by the body's normal defenses.

Downs hoped in 1939 to go to Paris to study at the Pasteur Institute. On sabbatical in New York, she studied French in preparation for the trip. World War II interrupted her plan, however, and in 1943 the government called her to work at its top-secret biological warfare research center at Fort Detrick in Frederick, Maryland.

Her work there is a blank; she published no papers until 1946. Her top-secret clearance made normal interactions difficult. When her department chair at Kansas wrote asking her to return for fall semester, she was unable even to tell him she could not come until he, too, had been issued clearance. At least some of her work seems to have involved tularemia, since the four papers she published in 1946 all dealt with the bacteria.

At the University of Kansas, Downs won a distinguished academic post created by a man who said no woman would ever deserve to hold it.

After the war Downs collaborated with Russian researchers, who had come up with a strain of *P tularensis* that looked promising for use in a human vaccine. From the Russian bacteria, Downs finally developed the strains that could be used for the human vaccine.

After the conclusion of her tularemia research, Downs worked during the late 1950s and early 1960s to develop a new staining technique. She found a stable compound that was effective in her technique and published her discovery in a much-heralded paper. "Isothiocyanate compounds as fluorescent labeling agents for immune serum," published in the *American Journal of Pathology* in 1958, was one of the one hundred most cited articles in the fifteen-year period between 1961 and 1974.

Downs officially retired at seventy in 1963, although she published a paper in 1970 and was appointed to the position of Sommerfield Distinguished Professor of Bacteriology at Kansas in 1972. (The chair's founder once said that no woman would ever win the position because no woman would ever deserve it).

In 1980 her local branch of the American Society of Microbiology voted to rename a graduate student award after her. She died in her Lawrence, Kansas, at the age of ninety-five.

TO FIND OUT MORE . . .

- O'Hern, Elizabeth Moot. *Profiles of Pioneer Women Scientists.* New York: Acropolis Books, 1985.
- Downs's papers are at the Schlesinger Library at Radcliffe College.

Helen Flanders Dunbar, 1902–1959

P sychiatrist Helen Flanders Dunbar kept reinventing herself. Her childhood, after the age of eleven, was somewhat lonely, so she turned her intensely focused mind to academics, proving herself a capable and versatile scholar of philosophy, divinity, and medicine. Before the age of thirty she had earned four advanced degrees, including a Ph.D. and a medical degree, and become a gregarious charmer with many ardent admirers.

Dunbar was born in Chicago to a patent attorney and mathematician, Francis William Dunbar, and a genealogist and translator, Edith Vaughan Flanders Dunbar. Dunbar and her younger brother Francis were very close, and when their father began to withdraw from the family, they spent much of their time together. They took private lessons from tutors and took trips to the Caribbean, California, and Central and South America.

Dunbar moved to New York City with her mother and brother, where she enrolled at the Brearley School for girls. At fifteen, she was short (4'11") and stout, and she felt she was an outcast among her peers. She poured her frustrated energy into her work, and propelled herself to incredible heights in a very short time. She attended Bryn Mawr College, graduating in 1923. From there she went on to graduate work in philosophy at Columbia University, earning a master's degree in 1924. She wrote her doctoral thesis on religious and scientific symbolism in *The Divine Comedy* by Dante Alighieri, grounding her work with a B.D. with honors from Union Theological Seminary. A year before she was awarded her Ph.D. in 1927, she enrolled at the Yale University School of Medicine.

Her last year of medical school was spent in Europe. She studied with Carl Jung in Zurich in her year abroad, returning in 1930 to accept her M.D. from Yale. On her return, she was the object of much attention from men, but in 1932 she married Ted Wolfe, a psychiatrist whom she had met in Zurich. The marriage lasted for seven years; the couple had no children. Dunbar kept her own name, which she had originally changed to H. Flanders Dunbar, then to Flanders Dunbar.

Dunbar's work followed its pattern of combining her many areas of knowledge. She united her knowledge of theology and psychology to direct, in 1930, the Council for the Clinical Training of Theological Students. The psychological training she was able to offer prospective ministers through the organization proved invaluable to their life work.

Before the age of thirty, Dunbar had earned four advanced degrees.

She combined psychology and medicine in her best-remembered work, an extensive study of psychosomatic factors in health. She identified a disturbed personality profile that was especially accident-prone, perhaps in an unconsciously self-destructive way. Her findings, published in her 1943 *Psychosomatic Diagnosis*, were extremely influential; in 1942 she founded the American Psychosomatic Society.

In 1939 Dunbar divorced Wolfe and almost immediately married *New Republic* editor George Henry Soule, Jr. They had one child, Marcia Dunbar-Soule, two years later, when Dunbar was nearly forty and Soule about fifty-five. Marcia became the focus of Dunbar's personal and professional life. She wrote popular books on child development, following the course of Marcia's growing up. She was unhappy with Soule, however, and lived for a time with a colleague, gynecologist Dr. Raymond Squier. She lived out her last eight years with Soule after Squier committed suicide in 1951.

A lawsuit by a former patient and alcohol abuse played their parts in her increasing depression, and in 1954 a disfiguring automobile accident further damaged her self-esteem. When her daughter found her drowned in the pool at her South Kent, Connecticut, home, the newspapers hinted darkly that her death could be a suicide, although there was no evidence to support that implication.

TO FIND OUT MORE . . .

- Sicherman, Barbara, and Carol Hurd Green, eds. *Notable American Women: The Modern Period. A Biographical Dictionary.* Cambridge, MA: The Belknap Press of Harvard University Press, 1980.

- Some of Dunbar's papers are at the Union Theological Seminary Library.

Ethel Collins Dunham, 1883-1969

Pediatrician Ethel Dunham made premature babies her special concern. Her research and publications on the high mortality rate of premature infants made her a leading figure in her field. She worked to establish special care for premature children, and supplemented her understanding of early development with field research on primates.

Dunham was the eldest of six children born to Samuel G. Dunham, a well-off businessman, and Alice Dunham, a quiet amateur painter. Ethel was born and raised in Hartford, Connecticut, where, after graduating from high school, she lived for a time as a genteel but idle young lady. She tired of the golf, European tours, and endless social activities at age twenty-six and reenrolled at Hartford High School to finish her college entrance requirements.

She earned her bachelor's degree from Bryn Mawr in 1914 and continued her schooling at Johns Hopkins Medical School.

Her friend and lifetime companion **Martha May Eliot**, eight years Dunham's junior and a friend from Bryn Mawr, enrolled with her at Hopkins. They were two of only eleven women in a class of nearly one hundred students. After graduation they shared a home until Ethel's death over five decades later, excepting a few years when their work took them to different cities.

After their graduation in 1918, the pair briefly split up to pursue internships and residencies at different hospitals, Dunham interning in pediatrics at Johns Hopkins. In 1920 they were reunited in New Haven, where both taught at Yale University's School of Medicine. Dunham was an organizing force within the pediatrics ward, troubleshooting scheduling problems and soothing conflicts between obstetricians and pediatricians in the nursery. Her easy manner and gently humorous approach made her a natural facilitator.

In 1927 Dunham was made the medical officer in charge of neonatal studies at the Children's Bureau. She conducted a study of mortality in 1,000 newborns, in which she found that the most significant cause of death was premature birth. She brought her findings to the American Pediatric Society in 1933; the organization responded by making her the chair of a committee on neonatal studies.

Dunham and Eliot moved to Washington, D.C., in 1935 to take the respective positions of director of the child development research division and assistant chief of the Children's Bureau. Dunham took the opportunity to develop hospital standards for the care of newborns (especially premature ones). In 1943, her pioneering *Standards and Recommendations for the Hospital Care of Newborn Infants, Full Term and Premature* was published. It was one of the Academy of Pediatrics' most widely distributed works.

After the publication of another of Dunham's books, *Premature Infants, a Manual for Physicians*, in 1948, Dunham and Eliot moved to Geneva, Switzerland. They spent two years working for the World Health Organization there before Eliot's appointment as chief of the Children's Bureau in 1951 brought them back to Washington. In the early 1950s Dunham began to study primate behavior at birth and in rearing young. She also proposed using the Virginia opossum as a model for the study of premature offspring.

In 1957 the two scientists moved to Cambridge, MA, where Eliot became a full professor at Harvard University. That same year, Dunham became the first woman to win the American Pediatric Society's highest honor, the Howland Medal. She died twelve years later of broncho-pneumonia at age eighty-six.

> *Dunham was a pioneering researcher in the field of premature birth.*

TO FIND OUT MORE . . .

- Sicherman, Barbara, and Carol Hurd Green, eds. *Notable American Women: The Modern Period. A Biographical Dictionary.* Cambridge, MA: The Belknap Press of Harvard University Press, 1980.
- Dunham's papers are in the Ethel Collins Dunham Collection and the Martha May Eliot Collection in the Schlesinger Library at Radcliffe College.

Alice Eastwood, 1859–1953

The botany collection at the California Academy of Sciences in San Francisco was Alice Eastwood's responsibility for fifty-seven years. She nurtured it with deep devotion, and when a fire consumed the Academy building in 1906, she acted to save many of the collection's irreplaceable specimens, leaving her own belongings for the fire.

Eastwood's childhood was not particularly conducive to scholarly achievement. She was born in Toronto, Canada, where her father was the steward of the Toronto Asylum for the Insane. She grew up on the grounds of the place until age six, when her mother died. Alice was then given over to the care of an uncle, who taught her Latin plant names. She lived in a convent, where she learned gardening, when she was between eight and fourteen years of age, and was finally reunited with her father and two younger siblings in Denver, Colorado.

Eastwood's education was understandably spotty, but her interest in plants dated from an early age and had been regularly encouraged by adults in her life. She brought her enthusiasm and quick mind to her classes in Denver and graduated valedictorian of her class in 1879. She stayed on at East Denver high to teach and pursue her botany hobby for the next decade. Her regular hikes in the Colorado mountains were her greatest joy, and she was able to resign from her teaching job in 1890 to tour California and Colorado. During this period she gathered material for a guidebook she published three years later, *Popular Flora of Denver, Colorado*.

In 1892 Eastwood was invited to take a post as an assistant at the California Academy of Sciences in San Francisco by its curator, Katherine Brandegee, an acquaintance from her travels. For $75 a month, she organized the Academy's collection and founded and directed the California Botanical Club. When Brandegee left in 1894, Eastwood took over her duties. She was extremely happy at the Academy—her job immersed her in her favorite subject and sent her on frequent collecting trips to different parts of North America. She made the Academy her home until her retirement in 1949.

The fire and earthquake of 1906 much depleted the Academy's collection, despite Eastwood's prompt actions in saving some specimens. Eastwood spent much of her career building the collection to new levels of excellence, collecting over 340,000 specimens, many from the Sierra Nevada and the Coast Ranges, that more than replaced those lost in the fire. She kept the Academy a cheerful and inviting place for visitors, exhibiting fresh and ever-changing displays of flowers in the foyer. She also published other guidebooks, several articles, and a journal, *Leaflets of Modern Botany*, in addition to her regular duties.

> *During San Francisco's 1906 earthquake and fire, Eastwood chose to save irreplacable botanical specimens rather than her own belongings.*

After her retirement she was asked to serve as the honorary president of the Seventh International Congress in Stockholm in 1950, where she had the pleasure of sitting in the chair of Carolus Linnaeus, the botanist who founded the modern system of classification for flora and fauna. She died three years later at age ninety-three.

TO FIND OUT MORE ...

- Dakin, Susanna Bryant. *Perennial Adventure: A Tribute to Alice Eastwood.* San Francisco: California Academy of Sciences, 1954

- Ogilve, Marilyn Bailey. *Women in Science.* Cambridge, MA: The MIT Press, 1986.

- Sicherman, Barbara, and Carol Hurd Green, eds. *Notable American Women: The Modern Period. A Biographical Dictionary.* Cambridge, MA: The Belknap Press of Harvard University Press, 1980.

- Wilson, Carol Green. *Alice Eastwood's Wonderland: The Adventures of a Botanist.* San Francisco: California Academy of Sciences, 1955.

Tilly Edinger, 1897–1967

Paleontologist Tilly Edinger was a pioneer in the field of paleoneurology. She used fossils to study the development of the brain in mammals, contributing significantly to the understanding of the workings of the brain and of evolution. She has been ranked among a handful of the top figures in international vertebrate paleontology—of both sexes—in the twentieth century.

Born Johanna Gabrielle Ottelie Edinger in Frankfurt am Main, Germany, she was the youngest of three children in a socially prominent family. Her mother was a philanthropist and reformer, and her father conducted groundbreaking medical research in the new field of comparative neurology. He was not supportive of Edinger's ambition to pursue a career in science, since, however, he thought professional work was unsuitable for women. Nevertheless she studied natural philosophy in Heidelberg, Munich, and Frankfurt, where she earned her Ph.D. in 1921, with a doctorate on the brain cavity of an extinct reptile, *Nothosaurus*.

She stayed in Frankfurt as a research assistant in paleontology until 1927, when she was made the curator of the vertebrate collection of the Senckenberg Museum in Frankfurt. The job offered practical experience but no pay. From this position she could, and did, publish. One of her most important contributions was *Fossil Brains* (*Die Fossilen Gehrine*), published in 1929.

As the political climate shifted in the thirties, Edinger found that her religion—she was Jewish—was getting in the way of her work. By 1933 it had gotten so bad that the museum director was obliged to make her employment at the museum a secret. She entered by a side door and her name was removed from the front door. A Frankfurt street named for her father was renamed and a bust in honor of her mother removed. In 1938 it was discovered that she was still working at the museum, and she was forced to flee to London. Much later she learned that her brother Fritz had not escaped in time. He died in a concentration camp.

In 1940 she settled permanently in Massachusetts, where she worked for the rest of her life at Harvard University's Museum of Comparative Zoology. 1948 was the year of the publication of her other major contribution to her science, *The Evolution of the Horse Brain*. Her findings in this work had implications that went far beyond the confines of paleoneurology. She showed that an enlarged forebrain evolved independently in several different groups, indicating that evolution in this case was not a linear process but a many-branched process of natural trial and error.

Within the field of paleoneurology, Edinger was a major pioneer. By closely studying casts of the inside of fossil skulls, she was able to observe changes in the structure of the outer layer of the brain. She was one of the first to see this fossil evidence as anything but a curiosity, and her work paved the way for other researchers in this field.

Edinger was partially deaf in her later years. She died after being hit by a car near her home in Cambridge.

> *Edinger, who was Jewish, was forced to work in secret at Frankfurt's Senckenberg Museum in the 1930s.*

- Edinger's records are at the Museum of Comparative Zoology at Harvard University, and the AAUW Foundation in Washington, D.C.

TO FIND OUT MORE . . .

- Obituary. *The New York Times*, May 29, 1967.

- Sicherman, Barbara, and Carol Hurd Green, eds. *Notable American Women: The Modern Period. A Biographical Dictionary.* Cambridge, MA: The Belknap Press of Harvard University Press, 1980.

Martha May Eliot, 1891–1978

. . . .

This pediatrician and researcher's work with the United States Children's Bureau spanned three decades and helped make her an internationally known expert on child health. Her extraordinary career took her to posts all over North America and in Europe.

Martha May Eliot was born on April 7, 1891, in Dorchester, Massachusetts. She went to college at Bryn Mawr for a year, but graduated from Radcliffe in 1913. At Bryn Mawr, she met **Ethel Dunham**, an older woman from a genteel background. They enrolled together at Johns Hopkins Medical School in 1914. The two medical students became very close and would spend their lives together, with the exception of a few years spent working in different locations, until Ethel's death fifty-five years later.

Eliot earned her M.D. in 1918 and left Johns Hopkins for an internship at the Peter Bent Brigham Hospital in Boston, Massachusetts. She spent some time working at a hospital in St. Louis before joining Dunham at the Yale University School of Medicine in New Haven, Connecticut, in 1920. Dunham was one of the New Haven Hospital's first house officers, and Eliot started out in the new pediatrics department. Eliot's fourteen-year teaching career at Yale began a year later, when she was hired as an instructor. In 1924 she began her long association with the United States Children's Bureau.

At Yale Eliot conducted research on the prevention and control of rickets, a disease caused by vitamin D deficiency. Rickets, which is characterized by defective bone growth, attacked primarily children before better knowledge of nutrition mostly wiped it out in North America. Eliot also made a major contribution to the literature on infants' health when she revised the government standard *Infant Care*. In the 1930s, however, Eliot's attention turned more and more to administrative work with the Children's Bureau.

In 1935 Eliot was made the assistant chief of the Bureau. She moved to Washington, D.C., with Dunham, who took a position as the director of the division of research in child development at the Children's Bureau. Her work there led her to ever-broader efforts to further the interests of children worldwide, and she helped to found two major international children's advocacy programs, the World Health Organization (WHO) and the United Nations International Children's Emergency Fund (UNICEF). In 1947 she became the first woman to be elected president of the American Public Health Association.

Eliot helped found both the World Health Organization and UNICEF.

Eliot and Dunham moved to Geneva in 1949, where Eliot held the post of Assistant Director-General of the World Health Organization for two years. They returned to Washington when Eliot was made the Children's Bureau's chief in 1951. After Eliot's retirement from the Bureau, the pair moved to Cambridge, Massachusetts in 1957. Eliot worked at Harvard University's School of Public Health for three years on the Visiting Committee before she became one of the few women then on the Harvard staff as full professors.

After retiring from her post as Professor of Maternal and Child Health, Eliot headed the Massachusetts Committee on Children and Youth. Under her leadership, the committee undertook several influential projects, including a study of the Massachusetts welfare system that led to new welfare laws. Dunham died in 1969, and Eliot retired the next year from her duties as director. She left her personal papers and a series of recorded interviews with the Schlesinger Library at Radcliffe College between 1969 and 1976. She died in 1978, in her eighty-seventh year.

TO FIND OUT MORE . . .

- Sicherman, Barbara, and Carol Hurd Green, eds. *Notable American Women: The Modern Period. A Biographical Dictionary.* Cambridge, MA: The Belknap Press of Harvard University Press, 1980.

- Eliot's papers are in the Martha May Eliot Collection in the Schlesinger Library at Radcliffe College.

Alice Catherine Evans, 1881–1975

I n 1917, while working for the government as a health researcher, Alice Evans discovered the cause of brucellosis, a sneaky bacteria carried in raw milk. Its symptoms aped those of other diseases, making it extremely hard to diagnose in humans. She recommended its cure—pasteurization—thirteen years before her findings were finally accepted and put into action. Later, musing on the possible reasons one prominent scientist may have had for ignoring her findings, she said, "The Nineteenth Amendment was not a part of the Constitution of the United States when the controversy began, and he was not accustomed to considering a scientific idea proposed by a woman."

Evans grew up in Pennsylvania, the daughter of Welsh parents. Alice went to nearby schools for her high school degree. On graduation she worked in rural schools as a teacher for four years; she used the scant amount she saved to go to Ithaca,

New York, to take a two-year course in nature study designed for teachers.

Evans earned her M.S. in bacteriology at the University of Wisconsin. Although a supportive professor urged her to take a scholarship in chemistry, she instead accepted another's offer of a research job working in bacteriology for the government. She began work immediately upon graduation.

Assigned to ferret out sources of bacterial contamination in dairy products, Evans spent her own time studying the bacteria present in uncontaminated pasteurized fresh milk, taken from healthy cows, which was then considered innocuous. She made a new connection between "Malta fever," caused in humans by a bacteria called *Micrococcus melitensis*, and spontaneous abortion in cows, caused by *Bacillus abortus*. Malta fever had been traced to goats' milk in 1887. *Bacillus abortus* had been isolated in 1897. Despite their different-sounding names, the two bacteria—and a third that had been recently discovered in pigs—looked and acted nearly identically in Evans' lab.

Evans drew the logical conclusion that what killed people when transmitted by goats might kill them just as easily when transmitted by cattle. In 1917 she presented her findings at a meeting of the Society of American Bacteriologists; in 1918, she published them in the *Journal of Infectious Diseases*. Her colleagues were doubtful; one eminent opponent, an acknowledged authority on both human and animal diseases, was outspoken in his opposition. The dairy industry was even less polite; her findings were a threat to their livelihood.

Evans retreated for a few years, switching her attention to influenza and meningitis. But at the end of World War I, she returned to her study of the group of milk-borne bacteria, demonstrating methodically that strains found all over the world belonged to a single family. In the course of her long unappreciated work, Evans actually contracted brucellosis from a goat-borne strain. She was plagued with the elusive, recurring symptoms for the next twenty-three years, until the introduction of antibiotics.

> **Evans' work was instrumental in forcing the dairy industry to pasteurize its milk.**

Slowly, more established scientists began to verify Evans' early findings. In 1920 a new genus, *Brucellus*, was proposed to cover the family. It wasn't until the early 1930s, however, that further studies documented cases of milk-transmitted brucellosis in humans, and overwhelming scientific opinion combined to force the dairy industry to pasteurize all milk sold in the United States.

Evans' work earned her recognition years after the fact. She was elected the first woman president of the Society of Bacteriologists in 1928; after her retirement at age 64 she was honored by the Inter-American Committee on Brucellosis and the American Society for Microbiology. She died in 1975 at the age of ninety-four.

TO FIND OUT MORE . . .

- O'Hern, Elizabeth Moot. *Profiles of Pioneer Women Scientists.* New York: Acropolis Books, 1985.

- Sicherman, Barbara, and Carol Hurd Green, eds. *Notable American Women: The Modern Period. A Biographical Dictionary.* Cambridge, MA: The Belknap Press of Harvard University Press, 1980

- Vare, Ethlie Ann, and Greg Ptacek. *Mothers of Invention: From the Bra to the Bomb, Forgotten Women and Their Unforgettable Ideas.* New York: William Morrow, 1988.

Matilda Arabella Evans, 1872–1935

. . . .

Surgeon and child advocate Matilda Evans worked in Columbia, South Carolina, where few medical facilities existed for the mostly impoverished African-American half of the city's population around the turn of the century. She single-handedly changed that dismal situation, founding free-care clinics, three hospitals, a nursing school, and a South Carolina health care organization. She changed government policy on child health care in public schools and on public sanitation. All this was accomplished while running her own busy practice and single-handedly raising seven adopted children.

Matilda Evans was born in Aiken, South Carolina. She attended the town's Schofield Industrial School, founded through the Pennsylvania Freedmen's Association by Martha Schofield of Philadelphia. The school was established to provide African-American children in South Carolina with a rigorous education. At the Schofield

school, Evans developed an ambition to become a medical missionary abroad. She earned a bachelor's degree from Oberlin College in 1891, working in the dining hall and at home in the summers to pay her way, and returned to Schofield to teach after a short teaching stint in Georgia.

With her meager teacher's salary, a $100 grant in her second year, and assistance from Martha Schofield, Evans earned her M.D. from the Woman's Medical College of Pennsylvania in 1897. Upon graduation she returned to become the first African-American woman to practice medicine in Columbia, South Carolina. Her services were in great demand, regardless of the color of her patients. While she planned more permanent health services for Columbia, she opened her own house as a hospital and ran a free clinic for infants.

When the young surgeon started her humanitarian work, Columbia's health care facilities were sadly inadequate. Evans set

72

out to patch up the holes. She founded the Columbia Clinic Association and visited established clinics in New York, Durham, and Philadelphia to gather ideas for the clinic the Association was planning. At first run out of a church basement, the popular service soon moved into permanent quarters. All services were free to the public. Its staff included a dentist and an eye, ear, nose and throat specialist, and it was able to provide free vaccinations for children and some mental health services.

Evans was particularly concerned about the poorer children of the area, and began to give examinations on her own time to the African-American public school students. She found many problems that showed a lack of medical attention: ringworm, scabies, decayed teeth, bad tonsils, untreated infections. She was able to document enough neglect to convince the public school system to implement a permanent program to provide students with regular examinations.

Other projects in Columbia founded by Matilda Evans included the Negro Health Care Association of South Carolina and the Taylor Lane Hospital and Training School

Evans documented enough health problems among poor black Southern children to force public schools to provide regular medical examinations.

for Nurses (later Saint Luke Hospital). The hospital was the only one in the area set up to serve African-American patients. Evans served as its superintendent, overseeing a staff of several physicians.

Evans was as generous with her personal time as she was with her professional work. She once taught herself to swim so that she could offer free swimming lessons to neighborhood children in a pond on her land. Her love of children led her to adopt seven of them, whom she raised alone (she never married). She died at her home at age sixty-three after a brief illness.

TO FIND OUT MORE . . .

- Caldwell, A.B., ed. *History of the American Negro* (South Carolina edition). Atlanta: A.B. Caldwell Co., 1919.

- Lerner, Gerda, ed. *Black Women in White America.* New York: Pantheon, 1972.

- Smith, Jessie Carey. *Notable Black American Women.* Detroit, MI: Gale Research Inc., 1992.

Margaret Clay Ferguson, 1863-1951

. . . .

Around the turn of the century, botany was considered a fine hobby for a woman. Many pursued it as a diversion. For Margaret Ferguson, however, it was serious work. She grounded her study of botany in chemistry and genetics and taught her Wellesley students to do the same, bringing to her field a new measure of scientific legitimacy.

Margaret Ferguson, the fourth of six children, was born in Orleans, New York. Her father was a farmer in nearby Phelps, New York. Margaret was a sharp student who began to teach at age fourteen in local public schools. While she taught, she took classes at Genesee Wesleyan Seminary in Lima, New York. At twenty-four she became an assistant principal. Three years later she was accepted at Wellesley College as a special student in botany and chemistry.

Ferguson spent two years (1891–1893) as head of the science department at Harcourt Place Seminary in Gambier, Ohio.

When the head of Wellesley's botany department asked her to return to Wellesley as an instructor, however she went gladly. She spent the rest of her career at Wellesley, excepting a five-year chunk she spent traveling and earning her Ph.D. at Cornell. Her graduate work at Cornell included a life history of a North American pine tree, a study that set a standard for other such studies.

When she returned to Wellesley in 1901, she was thirty-nine. She rose quickly through the academic ranks, moving from instructor to full professor in only five years. In 1902 she was made head of the botany department. She was a wonderful teacher who emphasized an interdisciplinary approach to her field, teaching her students the importance of chemistry, physics, and zoology in botany. She also stressed the importance of laboratory work, and decided that Wellesley's botany facilities needed improvement.

Over the course of almost thirty years

Ferguson had the Wellesley facilities rebuilt to her specifications. It was a colossal job, but Ferguson planned, designed, and raised the money for a complex of two greenhouses and an attached botany building. The new labs were made to allow Wellesley students to study genetics, a field that became more intriguing to Ferguson herself as the labs were being built.

In her sixties Ferguson took on an ambitious new project in genetics. She used plants of the genus *Petunia* as a tool for studying the genetics of higher plants. She straightened out the then-convoluted taxonomy of the *Petunia* group and reported that the gene pairs were unstable. Her conclusions, published in her 1924 article in *Anatomical Record*, were proven right almost fifty years later when technology caught up to her work.

> *Ferguson's observations on the taxonomy of a group of plants were a half century ahead of their time.*

Ferguson finally retired from Wellesley in 1938 at age seventy-five. She returned to New York State to be with her family. Before her 1951 death in San Diego, Wellesley College named the botany department's new greenhouses after her.

TO FIND OUT MORE...

- Hart, Sophie C. "Margaret Clay Ferguson." *Wellesley Magazine* (June 1932):pp. 408–10.

- Ogilve, Marilyn Bailey. *Women in Science: Antiquity through the Nineteenth Century*. Cambridge, MA: The MIT Press, 1986.

- Sicherman, Barbara, and Carol Hurd Green, eds. *Notable American Women: The Modern Period. A Biographical Dictionary*. Cambridge, MA: The Belknap Press of Harvard University Press, 1980.

Irmgard Flügge-Lotz, 1903–1974

Despite her anti-Nazi sentiments, engineer Irmgard Flügge-Lotz spent World War II working for Hermann Göring's aeronautics research institute. She made substantial contributions to aerodynamics, but was never able to secure a university position in the country of her birth. After the war, however, she moved to the United States, where she became the first woman professor of engineering at Stanford.

Irmgard was the child of a mathematician, Oscar Lotz, and Dora Lotz, the daughter of a family whose fortune had been made in construction. She often visited construction sites when she was young, and it was there that she developed her lifelong interest in how things worked.

She helped to pay her way through the Technische Hochschule in Hanover by working as a tutor in her spare time. There were few other women in her classes, which included fluid dynamics and applied mathematics. She loved her work; it seemed to her that engineering was a career in which she would never be bored. She earned her diploma in 1927 and stayed on to earn a Ph.D. in thermodynamics in 1929.

As a young research engineer at the Aerodynamische Versuchsanstalt at Göttingen, she worked with Ludwig Prandt, one of the founders of aerodynamics. She soon made her own mark. Before she was thirty, she had developed a new way to calculate the distribution, wingtip to wingtip, of the lifting force of a wing. Her method, called the Lotz method after her, worked even if the wings were not the same shape. She soon had her own research program at the institute.

In 1938 she married another engineer and a member of the faculty at Göttingen, Wilhem Flügge. Like her, he opposed the Nazi regime, and it had hampered his promotion at the University. That year, both engineers were hired—ironically—by Hermann Göring, who placed technical ability above politics in the all-important area of aerodynamics research. The Germans hoped to win the war with the technology, and they poured all available resources—including Wilhelm Flügge and Irmgard Flügge-Lotz—into the Deutsche Versuchsanstalt far Luftfahrt.

After the war, both researchers were asked to join the Office National d'Etudes et de Recherches Aeronautiques in Paris. They spent a year there before emigrating to the United States in 1948. Both secured positions at Stanford University, he as a full professor and she as a lecturer. She spent the rest of her professional career at Stanford, where she established graduate programs in mathematical aerodynamics and hydrodynamics. She published a major work on flight control systems for aircraft in 1953, *Discontinuous Automatic Control*, and became an American citizen in 1954.

In 1960 she was made a full professor, the first woman to gain that distinction in engineering at Stanford. In 1968 she published another work on aircraft control systems, was made a professor emerita, and retired. She was honored by the Society of Women Engineers and the American Institute of Aeronautics and Astronautics, and

Before she was thirty, Flügge-Lotz had developed a new way to calculate the distribution, wingtip to wingtip, of the lifting force of a wing.

continued to lecture and conduct research. She died after a long illness at the age of seventy-one.

TO FIND OUT MORE . . .

- Obituary. *The New York Times*, May 23, 1974.
- Sicherman, Barbara, and Carol Hurd Green, eds. *Notable American Women: The Modern Period. A Biographical Dictionary*. Cambridge, MA: The Belknap Press of Harvard University Press, 1980.

Martha Minerva Franklin, 1870–1968

In 1908, Martha Franklin decided that African-American nurses needed to band together to work to improve their status in their profession. She recruited over fifty nurses for the first meeting of the National Association of Colored Graduate Nurses (NACGN) that August, and served two terms as its president. Later, under the leadership of **Adah Thoms** during World War I, the NACGN integrated the Army Nurse Corps.

Martha Minerva Franklin was the middle of three children born to Henry and Mary Franklin. She grew up in Meriden, Connecticut, and attended public school. At twenty-five she moved to Philadelphia to enroll at the Woman's Hospital Training School there. Two years later she was the only African-American graduate in her class.

Franklin returned to Meriden, Connecticut, to work as a private nurse. Despite the fact that she was very fair and was often mistaken for white, she became increasingly aware that color was a major barrier in nursing. In 1906 she began to devote much of her spare time to studying the problem. Discovering that the obstacles she had run into were shared by most African-American nurses, she concluded that the group needed to work together to overcome them. She believed that a national organization would also gain them much-needed recognition from the public they served.

In 1908, fifteen hundred handwritten letters were sent out to nurses to organize the first meeting. Held at St. Mark's Methodist Episcopal Church in New York, the meeting attracted fifty-two members. The fledgling organization's goals were set: to wipe out bias in nursing, to promote leadership among African-American nurses, and to improve standards in both education and administration. Franklin was unanimously elected president, serving for two years before stepping down to make room for new leaders.

In 1912 the NACGN sent a representative to the International Council of Nurses meeting in Germany, integrating the older organization for the first time. By the end of World War I, the NACGN numbered over two thousand members; by 1940, over twelve thousand. Meanwhile, Franklin worked as a nurse in New York City and served as the organization's permanent historian and honorary president.

Franklin returned to school twice, once in 1920 to qualify as a registered nurse in New York and later at age fifty-eight to study public health nursing at Teachers' College at Columbia University. She eventually moved to New Haven to live with her older sister. She died there at ninety-eight years of age and was buried near her childhood home in Meriden, Connecticut.

> *Franklin recruited over fifty nurses for the first meeting of the National Association of Colored Nurses, and served two terms as its president.*

TO FIND OUT MORE . . .

- Carnegie, M.E. *The Path We Tread*. Philadelphia: Lippincott, 1986.

- Smith, Jessie Carey. *Notable Black American Women*. Detroit, MI: Gale Research Inc., 1992.

Virginia Kneeland Frantz, 1896–1967

· ·

Cancer researcher Virginia Kneeland Frantz was keenly aware of her position as a pioneering woman in medicine. Not only did she become a doctor in the 1920s, when few women thought of pursuing a career (much less a medical one), she chose to work in that most masculine of medical disciplines, surgery. She even considered rejecting the prestigious Elizabeth Blackwell Award for a woman who has made important contributions to medicine because she felt that it emphasized her gender, not her contributions. "I'm not a medical oddity," she protested.

Virginia Kneeland was the daughter of upper-class Manhattanites Yale and Anna Isley Ball Kneeland. She attended the exclusive and rigorous Brearley School for girls in New York City and Bryn Mawr College, where her exceptional aptitude in chemistry was noticed and encouraged. She graduated at the head of her class and took advantage of the new openings for women at the College of Physicians and Surgeons at Columbia University.

Although she was one of only five women in a class of seventy-four, she graduated second in her medical school class in 1922. In 1920 she married her classmate Angus MacDonald Frantz. In 1922 she became the first female doctor ever to undertake a surgical internship at the Columbia-affiliated Presbyterian Hospital in New York, gaining an appointment as an assistant surgeon and a member of the Columbia faculty in 1924. Meanwhile she had three children, Virginia (1924), Angus, Jr. (1927), and Andrew (1930), and tried to keep from stepping on her neurologist husband's professional toes by specializing in surgical pathology. Only five years after Andrew's tragically early death, however, the Frantzes were divorced.

Virginia Frantz had been a capable surgeon who belied the then-popular belief that women couldn't take the stress of surgical performance. As a researcher she was equally impressive. Her studies on breast cancer, thyroid cancer, and especially pancreatic tumors gained her national renown. She was one of the first, around 1940, to show that radioactive iodine was effective against thyroid cancer, and was a pioneer as well in studying chronic cystic disease in the breast. During the Second World War she discovered that oxidized cellulose could be used in a wound, where it controlled bleeding and was absorbed into the body. In 1948 she was given the Army-Navy Certificate of Appreciation for Civilian Service for her discovery.

Frantz rose steadily through the ranks at Columbia, becoming a full professor in 1951. She was an alert, challenging teacher who kept her students on their toes with her humor and quick eye. She was repeatedly honored by her peers, twice serving as the president of the New York Pathological Society (1949, 1950) and once as the first woman president of the American Thyroid Association (1961). After her retirement from Columbia in 1962, she continued to serve as a surgical consultant and kept an office at the Columbia-Presbyterian Medical Center.

Sadly, although she had done so much

Franz was one of the first researchers to demonstrate that radioactive iodine was effective against thyroid cancer.

to fight cancer, her research could not stop the cancer that killed her at age sixty-five. She died at home in 1967.

TO FIND OUT MORE ...

- *The National Cyclopedia of American Biography* L III, p. 346. New York: J.T. White.

- Obituary. *The New York Times,* Aug. 24, 1967.

- Sicherman, Barbara, and Carol Hurd Green, eds. *Notable American Women: The Modern Period. A Biographical Dictionary.* Cambridge, MA: The Belknap Press of Harvard University Press, 1980.

Else Frenkel-Brunswik, 1908–1958

Jewish-Austrian psychologist Else Frenkel-Brunswik left Vienna in 1938 after the *Anschluss* made her presence there dangerous. In America she studied anti-Semitic prejudice, publishing the classic study *The Authoritarian Personality* in 1950. As a Vienna-trained psychologist, she helped introduce American behaviorists to the nuances of psychoanalysis. Despite her brilliant professional successes, however, Frenkel-Brunswik's happiness was shattered in 1955 when her beloved husband, suffering terribly from severe hypertension, committed suicide. She overdosed on barbital three years later, at the age of forty-nine.

Else Frenkel was born in Poland, the daughter of Helene Gelernter Frenkel and bank owner Abraham Frenkel. When she was six, the family fled the 1914 pogrom, settling in Vienna. Else was a bright student who earned a Ph.D. in psychology at the University of Vienna at age 22. She stayed on, working as an assistant professor in psy-

chology, and only left in 1938 when political conditions made it impossible for her to stay.

She married Egon Brunswik, her psychology teacher. The fact that he was not Jewish was a problem for her family, but she was eventually forgiven by her father, to whom she was closest. They never had children, but loved each other deeply. She continued her research at Vienna and underwent psychoanalysis, laying the foundation for her later work in the United States. Egon had spent time at the University of California at Berkeley in 1937, and when the Nazis took over Austria in 1938, he had a position waiting for him in the United States.

The couple moved to California, where her husband had professorial status at Berkeley. Like so many talented scholars who happened to be married to other scholars, she had no opportunity to be considered for an academic position because of the standard rules against nepotism. Still, as a lecturer and a research psychologist, she was a tremendous asset to the university. Her considerable experience with psychoanalysis made her an authority on a subject still fairly foreign to American psychologists. She took an antinumerical stance against tests that sought to quantify every response, demonstrating that such tests could be misleading; subtler, more "speculative" tools, she stressed, should not be ignored.

In the 1940s she worked with three other researchers on an important study on prejudice. Her personal experiences with anti-Semitism added to her commitment to the project, which was underwritten by the American Jewish Committee in 1945. In 1950, *The Authoritarian Personality* was published, throwing off shock waves of reaction. Although the book was ardently lauded for its pioneering synthesis of social psychology and psychoanalysis and its carefully worked out model of the relationship between ideology and child raising, it was slammed by equally ardent critics.

Frenkel-Brunswik set about new studies on prejudice in children and on aging, but in 1955 she was devastated by her husband's suicide. His hypertension, despite depressive drug therapy and a corrective operation, had become intolerable to him. Frenkel-Brunswik never regained her equilibrium. She was awarded a Fulbright scholarship for study in Oslo and was made a full professor at Berkeley, but these honors were of no use to her at this late stage. She was found dead of an overdose of barbital in 1958.

> *Frenkel-Brunswik helped introduce American behaviorists to the nuances of psychoanalysis.*

TO FIND OUT MORE . . .

- Heiman, Nanette, and Joan Grant eds. *Else Frenkel-Brunswik: Selected Papers*, in *Psychological Issues*, VIII, Monograph 31 (1974).

- Sicherman, Barbara, and Carol Hurd Green, eds. *Notable American Women: The Modern Period. A Biographical Dictionary*. Cambridge, MA: The Belknap Press of Harvard University Press, 1980.

Frieda Fromm-Reichmann, 1889-1957

Psychoanalyst Frieda Fromm-Reichman is probably most popularly remembered as the doctor whose expert calm inspired Joanne Greenberg's (pen name Hannah Green) literary tribute to the healing power of a good psychoanalyst, *I Never Promised You a Rose Garden*. Fromm-Reichmann used her remarkable gifts as a psychiatrist and psychoanalyst to get through to many seriously disturbed patients like Greenberg. Her more quietly lasting contribution, however, was to get her colleagues to see, as she did, the unique individuals behind the barriers of schizophrenia and manic-depression.

Frieda Reichmann was born in Karlsruhe, Germany, and raised in Königsberg, East Prussia. Her mother, Klara, was an educated, forward-thinking woman who believed her three daughters should have an alternative to marriage. She organized private classes for them and for the daughters of other like-minded parents.

Reichmann was an excellent student and took her mother's opinion to heart. At the age of nineteen she enrolled at the medical school at Albertus University in Königsberg.

Reichmann was tiny—about four feet ten inches tall—and had a girlish appearance. Faculty members tended not to take her quite seriously, and she decided that obstetrics (her first ambition) would be difficult for a person of her size and strength. Instead, she turned to psychiatry, working from 1913 to 1918 at the university's psychiatric hospital. She supervised a one-hundred-bed hospital for soldiers with brain injuries near the end of World War I, and developed her natural compassion for patients so disturbed that verbal communication was all but impossible.

She was also psychoanalyzed herself in Munich and Berlin. The experience charged her with energy; she felt that psychoanalysis could cure the social evils of the world. She directed a private psychoanalytic hospital in

Heidelberg from 1924 until 1928. In 1926 she married a colleague at the hospital, social philosopher Erich Fromm. She was thirty-seven; he was twenty-six. The marriage broke up in the thirties.

When anti-Semitism began to make work difficult for her in the early thirties, Fromm-Reichmann left Germany. She spent time in France and Palestine, and finally settled in Maryland in 1935. She became a U.S. citizen in 1941. For the rest of her career her work was based at Chestnut Lodge, a private psychoanalytic sanitarium in Rockville, Maryland. She quickly rose to prominence among psychoanalysts, serving as the president of the Washington-Baltimore Psychoanalytic Society (1939–1940).

Her main interest was in deeply troubled, noncommunicative patients. These patients—often manic-depressives or schizophrenics—were not generally considered to be candidates for psychoanalysis, but Fromm-Reichmann brought her patience and sensitivity to her patients' sessions, listening carefully to the most garbled rantings or the most profound silence. Most of all, she was able to communicate to them that she was there, listening, and interested. To her colleagues she was an ardent advocate of her patients' individuality. She was especially interested in the link between creative genius and mental illness, and would use Van Gogh's painting, Robert Schumann's music, and Schopenhauer's writing to illustrate her point.

She continued to work up until her death. She received many honors in her later years, including a fellowship to Palo Alto at age sixty-six. She used it to examine nonverbal communication in psychotherapy. Ironically, this expert in the use of "the talking cure" lost her hearing in her later years. She died at Chestnut Lodge at the age of sixty-eight.

> *Fromm-Reichmann was an ardent advocate of the patient's individuality.*

TO FIND OUT MORE . . .

- Green, Hannah. "In Praise of My Doctor." *Contemporary Psychoanalysis* (Fall 1967).

- Marschak, Marianne. "One Year Among the Behavioral Scientists: In Memory of Frieda Fromm-Reichmann." *Psychiatry* (Aug. 1960).

- Sicherman, Barbara, and Carol Hurd Green, eds. *Notable American Women: The Modern Period. A Biographical Dictionary.* Cambridge, MA: The Belknap Press of Harvard University Press, 1980.

- Weigert, Edith. "In Memoriam: Frieda Fromm-Reichmann, 1889–1957." *Psychiatry* (Feb. 1958).

Julia Anna Gardner, 1882–1960

. . . .

Geologist Julia Anna Gardner lived through two world wars. In the first, moved by reports of the carnage in France, she served for two years in the Red Cross. During the second, however, she was able to put her expertise in invertebrate zoology to use to help defend against enemy bombs.

Julia Anna Gardner was the child of a doctor, Charles Henry Gardner, and his much younger second wife, Julia M. Brackett. The couple had no other children, and Julia's father died when she was still an infant, leaving her and her mother alone in Chamberlain, South Dakota. By the time she turned eight, her mother had moved with her back to her hometown of Dixon, Illinois. In 1898 they moved to North Adams, Massachusetts, and after Julia graduated they moved a third time to Vermont.

Julia's grandmother had left her a sum of money, and she used it to pay her way through Bryn Mawr College. The energetic head of the paleontology department at Bryn Mawr, **Florence Bascom**, became a mentor to Gardner. She stayed on at Bryn Mawr for her bachelor's degree, spent a year teaching grammar school, and returned for her master's degree in 1907. Bascom prompted her to continue her studies in paleontology, and in 1907 she enrolled in the doctoral program in paleontology at Johns Hopkins University.

She studied invertebrates at Hopkins and at the Woods Hole Marine Biological Laboratory. Her dissertation was written on fossils of molluscs, which became a lifelong interest. After earning her Ph.D. in 1911, she stayed at Hopkins, teaching and working as a research assistant (not always for pay). Gardner moved to Washington, D.C. to work for the United States Geological Survey (USGS) until 1917, when she went abroad to serve with the Red Cross in France. She was hurt in 1919, spent time in a hospital, and returned to the United States the next year.

Gardner moved to Texas to study Eocene invertebrates for the USGS Coastal Plain division, which rapidly promoted her from assistant geologist to associate geologist to geologist. She continued to work for the government through the twenties and thirties, switching to the Paleontology and Stratigraphy division when the Coastal Plain unit was dismantled.

During World War II, Gardner worked with the USGS Military Geology Unit. The unit helped the military by offering information gleaned from the smallest clues. One of Gardner's contributions was to identify the origin of some Japanese bombs. Small shells in the sand used as ballast could be used to identify the beaches that the sand—and hence the bomb—came from.

Gardner studied the geology of Japan and the Pacific Island after the war, mapping the area for the Office of the Chief of Engineers. She officially retired in 1952, but was almost immediately rehired by the USGS to continue work in the West Pacific. She also served for a year after her retirement as the president of the Paleontological Society, and the next year as the vice president of the Geological Society. Poor health, however, made it impossible for her to continue to work after 1954, and she died at home in Bethesda, Maryland, in 1960.

> *One of Gardner's contributions was to identify the origin of a number of Japanese bombs.*

TO FIND OUT MORE . . .

- Knopf, E.B. "Julia Gardner, A.B., M.A., '07." *Bryn Mawr Bulletin*, Winter 1961.

- Sicherman, Barbara, and Carol Hurd Green, eds. *Notable American Women: The Modern Period. A Biographical Dictionary*. Cambridge, MA: The Belknap Press of Harvard University Press, 1980.

- Gardner's professional papers are at the National Personnel Records Center, General Services Administration, St. Louis, MO; the Branch of Paleontology and Stratography, USGA, Washington, D.C.; and the Field Records Collection at the USGS Library in Denver, CO.

Hilda Geiringer, 1893-1973

Applied mathematician Hilda Geiringer was one of many Jewish scientists who fled Germany for the United States in the 1930s when Hitler came to power. Germany's loss was America's gain, and Geiringer taught and conducted research at Brown University, Bryn Mawr College, Wheaton College, and Harvard University. Although she never did return to live in Germany, she was recognized late in her career by her alma mater, the University of Vienna, and her employer until 1933, the University of Berlin.

Growing up in Vienna, Hilda Geiringer showed an early aptitude for mathematics. She had remarkable powers of memory, and loved mathematics as a high-schooler. Her parents were moderately well off—her father was a textile manufacturer—and were able to fund Hilda's education at the University of Vienna.

Geiringer started out on the theoretical side of her field, studying pure mathematics at Vienna. She earned her Ph.D. in 1917, writing a dissertation on double trigonometric series. *Trigonometrische Doppelreihen*

was published in 1918. Following a job editing the *Fortschritte der Mathematik*, she landed an academic job in applied mathematics, working as Richard von Mises' assistant at the University of Berlin. She never returned to pure mathematics.

In 1921, the same year she began work at Berlin, she married Felix Pollaczek, another mathematician. They had a daughter, Magda, the next year, but the marriage was a short one. By the time Magda was three, the couple was divorced. Magda stayed with her mother. After six years at Berlin, Geiringer was promoted to lecturer. She was recognized as an important asset to the university for her teaching as well as her contributions to research in plasticity theory and probability theory, but her eminence made no difference in 1933, when all Jewish educators at Berlin lost their jobs.

Geiringer and Magda (now eleven) fled to Turkey, where Geiringer learned Turkish to secure a position lecturing at Istanbul University. By 1939, even Turkey no longer seemed safe, and the Geiringers moved to the United States. In 1945 she became a

U.S. citizen. On her arrival in America, her English and her reputation were good enough to land her a position as a lecturer at Bryn Mawr College. She taught there until 1945.

In 1943 Geiringer was married to her former employer from the University of Berlin, Richard von Mises. Von Meises taught at Harvard, where he was a full professor, and Geiringer moved to Massachusetts to chair the mathematics department at Wheaton College in Norton, MA. In spite of the considerable administrative demands of her new job, Geiringer continued her research on her own time and saw her husband on the weekends.

> *Forced to flee Germany in 1933, Geiringer was honored by the University of Berlin in 1956.*

When von Mises died in 1953, Geiringer obtained a grant to finish his work at Harvard. In 1958, a year before her retirement from Wheaton (she still ran the math department), she published the completed *Mathematical Theory of Compressible Fluid Flow*. After her retirement she also revised some of his earlier works, smoothing out inconsistencies and tightening up his arguments. She continued to publish her own articles as well.

Overdue recognition came from Germany in the later years of her career. The University of Vienna honored the fiftieth anniversary of her graduation in 1967 with a special ceremony. And the University of Berlin, which had been ready to recognize Geiringer's accomplishments in 1933 when she was forced to leave, made her a professor emeritus with salary in 1956. She was honored by organizations in her adopted country as well, including Sigma Xi and the American Academy of the Arts and Sciences.

Geiringer was visiting her brother, a musicologist, in Santa Barbara, California when she died. She was six months short of her eightieth birthday.

TO FIND OUT MORE . . .

- Sicherman, Barbara, and Carol Hurd Green, eds. *Notable American Women: The Modern Period. A Biographical Dictionary*. Cambridge, MA: The Belknap Press of Harvard University Press, 1980.

- Geiringer's papers are in the Harvard University Archives at Harvard University and the Schlesinger Library at Radcliffe College.

Lillian Evelyn Moller Gilbreth, 1878–1972

In her extraordinarily long and accomplished life, Lillian Gilbreth was many things: an industrial engineer, a much-published author, a psychologist, and (certainly not least) a mother of twelve. She is most fondly remembered in the classic memoir *Cheaper by the Dozen* by two of her children, Ernestine and Frank, Jr.

Lillian was the first child of eight born to well-to-do William and Annie Moller in Oakland, California. Her mother was frail and often pregnant, and the little girl was mostly responsible for her younger siblings by age 13. She was a good student, and when she decided to study literature at the University of California at Berkeley, her parents supported her. On her graduation in 1900, she became Berkeley's first female Commencement Day speaker.

Moller spent an unhappy period at Columbia University, studying for her master's degree in English literature. She soon returned to Berkeley to complete the degree.

She was about to leave on a tour of Europe as a break from her doctoral studies in California when she met Frank Bunker Gilbreth, one of Boston's foremost building contractors. They were married in 1904 and moved together to New York.

Over seventeen years, the Gilbreths had twelve children. Lillian joined Frank in his work, becoming a partner in his new motion study business. Frank Gilbreth, who started as a bricklayer, had made his name by developing a method called "speed building." His new business worked to find the "one best way" to perform any task in industry, that is, the way requiring the least time and exertion. The growing Gilbreth clan moved to Providence, Rhode Island, in 1910, where Frank worked as a management consultant and Lillian earned a Ph.D. in psychology at Brown University.

Lillian published her book *Psychology of Management* in 1914. Over the next decade, she and Frank often lectured at business and engineering schools as pioneers in the field of motion study. They co-authored several books over the next ten years, mostly motion study textbooks. When Frank died in 1924, Lillian found that their contractors were not terribly enthusiastic about paying Lillian alone. Most of the Gilbreths' contracts were canceled, and Lillian found herself in the position of having to provide for twelve children without help.

Gilbreth applied her knowledge of motion study to home economics and published *The Home-Maker and Her Job* in 1929. She established a reputation for herself as a consultant to home economics departments at several universities, and wrote articles for women's magazines on housekeeping. She put all twelve children through college with her publications, lectures, and consulting work.

Long after her children were provided for, Gilbreth continued her research in engineering. She developed new methods for handicapped people to accomplish simple tasks and was called on to advise government organizations including the Civil Defense Advisory Commission (in 1951) and the Office of War Information (during World War II). She was honored by the Society of Industrial Engineers in 1921, although it did not then admit women members. In 1966, she was the first woman awarded the Hoover Medal for distinguished public service by an engineer. After her death of a stroke at ninety-three, the Society of Women Engineers created a fellowship in her memory

> *Gilbreth developed new methods for handicapped people to accomplish everyday tasks.*

TO FIND OUT MORE . . .

- Gilbreth, Frank Jr., and Ernestine Gilbreth Carey. *Cheaper by the Dozen.* New York: T.Y. Crowell, 1948.

- Sicherman, Barbara, and Carol Hurd Green, eds. *Notable American Women: The Modern Period. A Biographical Dictionary.* Cambridge, MA: The Belknap Press of Harvard University Press, 1980.

- Yost, Edna. *Frank and Lillian Gilbreth: Partners for Life.* New Brunswick, NJ: Rutgers University Press, 1949.

Hetty Goldman, 1881–1972

I n 1911, the energetic archaeology student Hetty Goldman became one of the first women to lead an archeological dig. She spent much of her career as an archaeologist working on excavations in Greece and Turkey. She was also a dedicated humanitarian who volunteered as a nurse in the Balkan Wars and who directed German refugees fleeing the Nazi regime during World War II.

Julius and Sarah Goldman, New Yorkers of German-Jewish descent, had four children. Hetty was the third. She grew up in comfort; her grandfather was a founder of the investment bank Goldman, Sachs and Co., and her father was a lawyer in the city. Hetty's uncle, a classicist, first piqued her interest in archaeology.

Goldman studied Greek and English at Bryn Mawr College, graduating with an A.B. in 1903. She returned to New York, dividing her time between work as a manuscript reader at a publishing house, the Macmillan Company, and graduate classes in Greek at Columbia University. In 1909, she chose academia over literature and enrolled at Radcliffe College to do graduate work in classics and archaeology.

An article she wrote while earning her master's degree, "The *Orestia* of Aeschylus as Illustrated by Greek Vase-Painting" made her the first woman awarded the Charles Eliot Norton fellowship to attend the American School of Classical Studies at Athens. During her two years there, she led her first dig at Halae, a small town in central Greece. The excavation uncovered some of the earliest traces of Neolithic village occupation. Goldman wrote her doctoral dissertation on terracotta remnants in Halae, receiving her Ph.D. from Radcliffe in 1916.

Goldman's research at Halae was punctuated by periods of volunteer work during the Balkan war and, immediately afterward, World War I. After several years spent working for the New York City Red Cross, Goldman returned to Greece. In 1922 she directed another dig, this time in ancient Ionia for Harvard's Fogg Museum. This excavation was cut short by the Graeco-Turkish War later the same year.

In 1924 Goldman became director of

excavations for the Fogg. More excavations followed in Turkey and Greece. Goldman's specialty was prehistoric life in Greece and Turkey, but the war-torn sites of her work often made it difficult for her to dig deeply in any one area for long periods of time. A successful excavation at Tarsus, in which the team had dug down to levels laid around 3000 B.C., was interrupted in 1936 by political unrest.

Goldman returned to the United States, where Princeton University made her its first woman professor at the Institute for Advanced Study. At Princeton she wrote up her Tarsus findings for publication and sponsored German refugees. After the war she was able to return to Tarsus, where the excavation was completed two years later. She retired to continue to write up the Tarsus research, publishing her conclusions in three volumes: *Excavations at Göslü Kule, Tarsus* (1950, 1956, 1963). In 1966 she was awarded the gold medal for Distinguished Archaeological Achievement from the AIA. She died in 1972, at the age of ninety.

> *A respected archaeologist, Goldman was also a dedicated humanitarian during times of war.*

TO FIND OUT MORE . . .

- Read, Phyllis J., and Bernard L Witleib. *The Book of Women's Firsts.* New York: Random House, 1992.

- Sichelman, Barbara, and Carol Hurd Green, eds. *Notable American Women: The Modern Period. A Biographical Dictionary.* Cambridge, MA: The Belknap Press of Harvard University Press, 1980.

- Weinberg, Saul, ed. *The Aegean and the Near East.* Locust Valley, NY: J.J. Augustin, 1956.

- Goldman's papers are at the Schlesinger Library at Radcliffe College.

Winifred Goldring, 1888–1971

The paleontologist Winifred Goldring once wrote that she had never married because she had not "as yet found anyone more attractive than my work." Yet few other women found paleontology attractive at the time; it was a field mostly empty of women. When Goldring was appointed New York's State Paleontologist in 1939, she was the first woman to hold the post. Her presidency of the Paleontological Society in 1949 was another such "first."

The fourth of eight daughters born to Frederick Goldring and Mary Grey Goldring, Winifred grew up surrounded by the beautiful Albany countryside and her father's flowers (he was a florist and maintained the orchid collection at the Erastus Corning Estate). Valedictorian of her high school class, Goldring was elected to Phi Beta Kappa and made a Durant Scholar in her senior and junior years at Wellesley College. After graduating in 1909, she stayed on at Wellesley as an assistant to geology professor Elizabeth F. Fisher, earning an A.M. there in 1912.

Goldring pursued further training for the next few years, teaching petrology and geology at Wellesley and taking classes at Columbia and, later, Johns Hopkins. In 1914, she returned to Albany, where she met and was hired by John M. Clarke, director of the New York State Museum. She was taken on as a "scientific expert" in the Hall of Invertebrate Paleontology, where she developed exhibits and researched mid-Paleozoic crinoids, a group of echinoderms including sea lilies and feather stars.

Goldring's work looking for the "missing link" between algae and vascular plants made her an authority in her field and the Albany museum's plant collection one of the world's best. Her exhibits were much praised as models of educational museum work, and gained her a reputation as an educator that proved useful in the publication of her textbook on fossils, published in 1929. She found herself quite content in the museum environment, and after a year at Johns Hopkins in 1921, never pursued an academic position.

Although she was well known and respected in her field, Goldring was turned down for a position with the United States Geological Survey in 1928 because, she was told, the Survey wanted a "he-man" paleontologist. She also noted that her salary was not on a par with those of her male colleagues. She was always determined not to let her gender limit her fieldwork, however. She learned to shoot a revolver and had a walking outfit with "bloomers" designed in order to maintain her independence.

> *Goldring searched for the "missing link" between algae and vascular plants.*

Goldring retired in 1955 at age sixty-seven; she had a tendency to overwork and had once pushed herself to the point of nervous collapse. She withdrew entirely from scientific work and relaxed in her Albany home, surrounded by her family. She died sixteen years later, two days before her eighty-third birthday.

TO FIND OUT MORE ...

- Fisher, Donald W. *Memorial to Winifred Goldring, 1888-1971.* Geological Soc. of America, November 1971.

- Read, Phyllis J., and Bernard L. Witleib. *The Book of Women's Firsts.* New York: Random House, 1992

- Sicherman, Barbara, and Carol Hurd Green, eds. *Notable American Women: The Modern Period. A Biographical Dictionary.* Cambridge, MA: The Belknap Press of Harvard University Press, 1980.

Grace Arabell Goldsmith, 1904-1975

. . . .

The multitalented physician and nutritionist Grace Goldsmith was a dancer before she decided on a career in medicine. As a physician she took a particular interest in the relationship between diet and health, working to educate the public about deficiency-related diseases like pellagra. In the 1940s she established the first nutrition training for medical students at her alma mater, Tulane University.

Arthur William and Arabell Coleman Goldsmith's only child, Grace, was born in St, Paul, Minnesota in 1904. She was an energetic young woman, an athlete and a dancer. She attended the University of Minnesota, then transferred to the University of Wisconsin, graduating with a B.S. in 1925. She was the physical education director of the New Orleans YWCA when a friend convinced her to try medical school.

Grace Goldsmith worked her way through medical school at Tulane University, teaching dance classes at the YWCA to pay her tuition. Nevertheless, she graduated at the top of her class, beating out the other five women and 102 men who graduated that year. She worked as an intern at New Orleans' Touro Infirmary for a year, then landed a position as a fellow in internal medicine at the Mayo Clinic in Rochester, Minnesota, in 1933. She published her first of over 105 articles in 1934, on pain related to heart disease. And in 1936, she returned to Tulane to teach, with an M.S. in medicine from the University of Minnesota.

At Tulane she pursued her interest in vitamin deficiency diseases, then a problem in New Orleans. Malnutrition, Goldsmith saw, took a needless toll among poorer patients. She energetically set about establishing tests for vitamin C deficiency and researching pellagra. She helped to institute recommended dietary allowances for niacin, the vitamin that prevents pellagra, and conducted other research on riboflavin, folic acid, and vitamin B12. She became a passionate public health educator and began to tout the benefits of nutritional enrichment of certain foods.

Nutrition problems in Louisiana led Goldsmith to consider the far larger problem worldwide. She conducted studies of populations in Newfoundland in the 1940s, exploring the effects of vitamin enrichment of foods. She was aware of the massive problem of world hunger, and marshaled her considerable talents to fight it by founding Tulane's nutrition training for medical students, a program that grew into the Tulane School of Public Health and Tropical Medicine. She was appointed its dean when it became a separate entity in the 1960s, becoming the first woman dean of a school of public health in the United States.

> *Goldsmith, a talented dancer, taught dance classes at the local YMCA to pay for medical school.*

Goldsmith was given the AMA's Goldberger Award in Clinical Nutrition in 1964. She served as the president of the American Institute of Nutrition (1965), the American Board of Nutrition (1966–67), and the American Society for Clinical Nutrition (1972–1973). She died in New Orleans at age 71.

TO FIND OUT MORE . . .

- Read, Phyllis J., and Bernard L. Witleib. *The Book of Women's Firsts.* New York: Random House, 1992

- Sicherman, Barbara, and Carol Hurd Green, eds. *Notable American Women: The Modern Period. A Biographical Dictionary.* Cambridge, MA: The Belknap Press of Harvard University Press, 1980.

Florence Laura Goodenough, 1886–1959

. . . .

Developmental psychologist Florence Goodenough didn't set out to become a psychologist. For eleven years she taught young students in small rural schools near her hometown of Honesdale, Pennsylvania. In her thirties, however, she brought her trained sensitivity to children to the field of psychology, and quickly established herself as an inventive theorist and a careful researcher.

Goodenough grew up on a farm in Honesdale, Pennsylvania, the youngest of eight children born to Lines and Alice Goodenough. She attended a local school and earned a bachelor's degree in teaching in 1908. She spent more than a decade teaching in small provincial Pennsylvania schools like the one she had attended.

When Goodenough was thirty-three, she moved to New Jersey to teach in public schools in Rutherford and Perth Amboy. At the same time she attended classes at Columbia University, earning a bachelor's degree in 1920 and a master's in 1921. After earning her master's degree, she switched to Stanford University in California to finish work on her Ph.D.

Her thesis was written on an intelligence test she had designed. Her subjects, children from three to thirteen years old, were asked to draw a man. Goodenough theorized that a child's level of development could be observed in the complexity and organization (not necessarily the skill) of a drawing of an everyday object. The thesis, *Measurement of Intelligence by Drawings*, was published in 1926, and Goodenough's test was widely used.

After earning her doctorate in 1924, Goodenough took a position as the chief psychologist at the Minneapolis Child Guidance Clinic. In 1926 she was appointed to the faculty at the University of Minnesota. In her research work with graduate students (she quickly gained the rank of research professor), she tackled a wide range of problems, mostly in the field of child development. She published two impressive works in 1931, *Experimental Child Study* (with John E. Anderson) and *Anger in Young Children*. In both, she paid close attention to the methods used in evaluating children.

Her interest in methodology put her on the cutting edge of psychological research in the 1930s and 1940s, when researchers were up in arms over the issue of intelligence tests. In 1932 she created the Minnesota Preschool Scale, which estimated intelligence in young children. She revised it in 1940 and 1942, and (also in 1942) wrote *The Mental Growth of Children from Two to Fourteen Years*, with Katherine Maurer.

Goodenough also created a test for adults during World War II. The test, designed for the officer-selection process of the Women's Army Corps, was a free-association test that used words with multiple meanings. Subjects were asked to give a brief response to each word. Results were evaluated based on the meaning of the word the subject chose. Unfortunately, her work on this test was cut short by her diabetes, which increasingly plagued her in later years. She was forced to retire from the Minnesota staff at the age of sixty.

The diabetes took most of her sight, and she was quite deaf, but Goodenough still had quite a bit to say. With the help of Lois M. Rynkiewicz, her niece, she published *Exceptional Children* in 1956. Her third revision of her classic *Developmental Psychology* was published in 1959, the same year that she died of a stroke in Lakeland, Florida.

A former teacher, Goodenough developed important tests measuring the intelligence of young children.

TO FIND OUT MORE . . .

- Harris, Dale B. (Obituary). *Child Development* 30 (1959): 305–6.

- Sicherman, Barbara, and Carol Hurd Green, eds. *Notable American Women: The Modern Period. A Biographical Dictionary.* Cambridge, MA: The Belknap Press of Harvard University Press, 1980.

- Goodenough's papers are in the Archives at the University of Michigan and in the files of the Institute of Child Welfare.

Bette Nesmith Graham, 1924–1980

Although she was no trained scientist, Bette Nesmith Graham's invention has been a boon to many. As a single mother (and an imperfect typist) working as a secretary in the fifties, she began to sneak a little pot of white paint into her desk. The paint—later marketed as Liquid Paper—covered her mistakes.

Bette Claire McMurray was born in Dallas to a car salesman and a housewife with an interest in painting. She was an impatient student; she dropped out of school at seventeen and married her high school sweetheart, Warren Nesmith, at eighteen. At nineteen she was a single mother—Warren was off fighting in World War II.

She was able to find a position as a secretary despite her lack of office skills, and learned to type on the job. She was adept enough at learning them to move slowly up the secretarial ladder, supporting herself and her son Michael on the income. Soon after Warren returned from service,

the Nesmiths were divorced, and she and Michael were on their own.

She was an executive secretary at Texas Bank & Trust when her makeshift typing skills caught up with her. The IBM carbon film ribbons that were in use at the time made it almost impossible to erase an error; they smeared messily and broadcast mistakes. Graham took an idea from a weekend job painting holiday windows: covering a mistake with paint instead of trying to rub it out. She began to smuggle white tempera paint into the office.

One boss grumbled about "that white stuff," and some secretaries considered it cheating, but her co-workers begged her for a little of her formula. The little business that developed out of her kitchen, first under the name "Mistake Out" and then under "Liquid Paper," boomed. Graham decided to take advantage of the demand for her idea. She began to teach herself a little chemistry in order to improve and patent the formula.

Graham consulted a chemistry teacher at her son's school, a worker at a paint manufacturing company, and library texts. She worked in her kitchen to make the fluid smooth, opaque, and quick to dry. When she was satisfied with the results, she applied for a patent. IBM turned down her proposal that they market her product, so she set out to market it herself.

Liquid Paper took a while to catch on nationally. It was a local business for almost ten years; Graham's son Michael, who helped her fill the bottles in the garage for the early years of the business, made it big as a TV star on the sitcom "The Monkees" before his mother's business took off. By 1968, however, Liquid Paper was a household word, and Graham didn't need her secretarial job anymore.

Bette Graham sold Liquid Paper to the Gillette Corporation in 1979 for $47.5 million, plus royalties. She spent the last years of her life working for various charities, and she willed her fortune equally to them and to her son.

> Graham sold her invention to Gillette in 1979 for $47.5 million—plus royalties.

TO FIND OUT MORE...

■ Vare, Ethlie Ann, and Greg Ptacek. *Mothers of Invention: From the Bra to the Bomb, Forgotten Women and Their Unforgettable Ideas.* New York: William Morrow, 1988.

Alice Hamilton, 1869–1970

Toxicologist Alice Hamilton was a major force in improving industrial safety standards in the early twentieth century. As a resident of Hull House, the famous Chicago social service center founded by Jane Addams, she came into contact with factory workers suffering from the toxic effects of the hazardous materials they worked with. What she saw goaded her into action.

Alice, the second of five children, was born in New York City and grew up on her father's family estate in Fort Wayne, Indiana. His influential family had secured him a position as a partner in a grocery store, and he was quite satisfied with his cushioned position until the business failed, when Alice was 16. Alice's mother maintained her independence within her husband's family and encouraged her children's aspirations despite their paternal relatives' conservatism.

Alice Hamilton attended the exclusive Miss Porter's School in Connecticut, and deciding to pursue a career that would allow her some independence, studied science at Fort Wayne School of Medicine and medi-

cine at the University of Michigan. She interned in Minneapolis and Boston from 1893 to 1894 and studied bacteriology and pathology in Ann Arbor, Johns Hopkins, and Leipzig. She found Germany offensive, citing its anti-Semitism and "woman-despising." She finally took her first job in 1897, as a professor of pathology at the Woman's Medical School of Northwestern University.

She moved into Hull House, where she was exposed for the first time to radical politics and poverty. Taking on the activist life of the house, she taught classes, acted as a surrogate older sister to children, and established a well-baby clinic. She was soon overwhelmed with the tension between her research and the enormous demands she could never hope to meet at Hull House, but she pressed on in a dedicated attempt to do her bit.

Ten years later, still struggling at Hull House, Hamilton's attention was drawn to the diseases of the "dangerous trades," or industrial jobs. Her social conscience shocked by the abuses of human life endemic to American labor in the early part of the century, she poured herself with new energy into fighting the system.

As supervisor of Illinois's state survey of industrial toxins, she began to document cases of lead poisoning. Her 1910 study implicated seventy-seven industrial processes in the poisoning of nearly six hundred workers. New Illinois regulations requiring regular testing and new safety measures were a direct result of her work.

Hamilton's tiny, fragile-looking frame belied her personal charisma. When she brought the entire force of her personality to bear on factory owners, she was often able to persuade the surprised businessmen to improve safety standards before they were coerced to do so by new regulations. Her strong personality would help her at Harvard Medical School, where in the early 1920s she became the first woman professor hired by the university. As an assistant professor of industrial medicine, she was most useful as a facilitator, raising funds for field studies and working with government, reform, and labor groups.

Hamilton spent two terms on the League of Nations' Health Committee (1924-1930) and visited Europe in the 1920s and 1930s. She was forced to retire from Harvard at sixty-six, but continued to work as a consultant in the Division of Labor Standards and as president of the National Consumers' League. She retired to Hadlyme, Connecticut, with her sister and published her autobiography, *Exploring the Dangerous Trades*, in 1943. She remained politically active into her eighties, writing letters to editors and congressmen, and died quietly of a stroke at 101.

> *Hamilton was often able to persuade factory owners to improve safety standards before new regulations required them to do so.*

TO FIND OUT MORE . . .

- Hamilton, Alice. *Ezploring the Dangerous Trades*. Boston, MA: Northeastern University Press, 1943.

- Sicherman, Barbara, and Carol Hurd Green, eds. *Notable American Women: The Modern Period. A Biographical Dictionary*. Cambridge, MA: The Belknap Press of Harvard University Press, 1980.

- Yost, Edna. *American Women of Science*. New York: J.B. Lippincott Company, 1955.

Ethel Browne Harvey,
1885–1965

· ·

Ethel Browne Harvey was a cytologist, or cell biologist, whose research made major strides toward answering the fundamental question of how a small cluster of cells grows into a living being. Despite the pioneering quality of her work, however, Harvey had no regular academic position and so had to rely on grants and fellowships, or her own resources, to conduct her research. Despite this handicap, she not only made solid scientific contributions but raised two boys at the same time.

Ethel Browne was the youngest of five children of an old, prominent Baltimore family. Her father was a practicing obstetrician-gynecologist and surgeon and a professor of gynecology at the Woman's Medical College of Baltimore. Both parents supported professional careers for women, and all three Browne daughters went to the preparatory Bryn Mawr School before college. On her graduation in 1902, she enrolled at the Woman's College of Baltimore (later renamed Goucher College).

After her graduation from Goucher, Browne decided to continue her education at Columbia University, studying cell biology. (Her two older sisters became doctors.) She began her lifelong study of the processes of embryo development at Columbia, writing a doctoral thesis on male germ cells of *Notonecta* (a genus of aquatic insects). The thesis was published in 1913, the year she earned her Ph.D. Women's academic groups recognized her with fellowships before and after her graduation, but she also supported herself by teaching high school science and math at girls' schools and by working as a laboratory assistant.

In 1916 Browne married a Princeton biology professor, Edmund Newton Harvey. Their two sons were born in 1916 and 1922. Ethel Harvey continued to work, hiring maids and governesses to help with the children. She conducted research in the United

States and abroad, working at labs in Bermuda and Japan, in North Carolina and California. She had a three-year position at New York University as an instructor in biology from 1928 to 1931. For most of her career, however, she worked without title or salary at Princeton during the school year, and at the Woods Hole Marine Biology Laboratory on Cape Cod during the summers.

Over her long career, which lasted into her late seventies, Ethel Harvey published about a hundred papers in various scientific journals. One of the better known of these was "Parthenogenetic Merogony of Cleavage without Nuclei in *Arbacia punctulata*," published in *Biological Bulletin* (1936). The cell nucleus was generally supposed to be the part of the cell that "directed" cell division and embryo development. Working with sea urchin eggs, Harvey discovered that the nuclei could be removed from the cells and they would still divide in concentrated sea water. Furthermore, the new cells would live for up to a month.

Based on these findings, Harvey hypothesized that cell division might be controlled by parts of the cell other than the nucleus. The genes in the nucleus, she proposed, directed later developments in the growing embryo. The mainstream press made much of her findings; articles on her findings appeared in *Time, Newsweek*, and *Life* in late 1937.

Harvey continued to work late into her seventies. She saw her sons grow up to enter careers in medicine and chemistry, and in her later years was recognized for her contributions. She was made a trustee of the laboratory at Woods Hole and a fellow of the American Association for the Advancement of Science. She died ten minutes away from Woods Hole, in Falmouth, in 1965.

> **For most of her career, Harvey worked without title or salary at Princeton.**

TO FIND OUT MORE . . .

- Sicherman, Barbara, and Carol Hurd Green, eds. *Notable American Women: The Modern Period. A Biographical Dictionary.* Cambridge, MA: The Belknap Press of Harvard University Press, 1980.

- Obituary. The *New York Times,* Sept. 3, 1965.

- Harvey's papers are in the Marine Biological Laboratory Library in Woods Hole, MA.

Harriet Boyd Hawes, 1871–1945

. . . .

In 1900, the archaeology student Harriet Boyd Hawes became the first woman to lead an archeological dig. She found an Iron Age tomb site at Kavousi, on the Grecian island of Crete. Her findings at her second dig in Gournia, the site of an ancient city on Crete, represented another kind of archaeological breakthough; it was one of the first small towns (as opposed to grand fortresses) found on the island.

Harriet Boyd was the fifth and youngest of the family. Her mother died soon after she was born, and she attached herself to her older brother, who was her "idol"—her words. He died young, but not before his love of ancient history, which he studied at Harvard, had been absorbed by his baby sister.

She spent four years teaching classics to private students from 1892 to 1896 before she made a daring move for a genteel young woman, traveling to Athens, Greece, to study at the American School of Classical Studies. During the Greco-Turkish War in 1897, Boyd served as a volunteer nurse and was awarded the Red Cross by the Queen of Greece. She spent four years at the American School, winning a fellowship in her last year there.

After her graduation in 1900, Boyd enthusiastically headed for Crete to get her hands really dirty with some field work. It was a good time to excavate in Crete, since the Ottomans had recently been overthrown and the area was now more hospitable to archaeologists. She spent a short time exploring Crete via mule with another young student from Boston, Jean Patten, and decided to dig at Kavousi in May. Her thesis on the Iron Age tombs she found there earned her a master's degree from Smith in 1901.

Smith hired Boyd in 1900 as an instructor, and she spent six years there teaching Greek and archeology. Her time at Smith was broken up by her regular trips back to

Greece, where she led a series of excavations at Gournia in 1901, 1903, and 1904. Directing the excavations was an enormous task involving the management of hundreds of workers and, later, the many artifacts she unearthed. In a time when Cretan archeology was at its height, Boyd was the first archeologist to discover and excavate an early Bronze Age Minoan town. Her find was especially valuable because the town was a small, humble one quite different from the elaborate palaces then being explored by other archaeologists.

Boyd's findings were embraced by the archeological community. She published them with the American Exploration Society in 1908 in a paper that is still considered a definitive study. The Archaeological Institute of America funded her national lecture tour in 1902.

She left Smith in 1906, marrying a British archaeologist she had met in Crete, Charles Henry Hawes. Their two children, Alexander and Mary, were born in 1906 and 1910. In 1909 the Boyds published a popular handbook, *Crete: The Forerunner of Greece.* Over the next decade, Harriet Hawes turned her attention to her family and her public service work. She established and ran a Smith College nursing program in France in 1917.

> **Boyd was the first archeologist to discover and excavate an early Bronze Age Minoan town.**

In 1919 Charles Hawes became assistant Director of the Museum of Fine Arts in Boston, and Harriet began lecturing again, teaching a course on Pre-Christian art at Wellesley College. She kept up her activity for causes she deemed worthy, and in 1933 was sued for $100,000 by a shoe company whose striking employees she had supported, perhaps a little too effectively. After sixteen years lecturing at Wellesley, she retired in 1936 with her husband to a farm in Alexandria, Virginia.

When Charles died, Harriet Hawes moved into a nearby rest home. She died there in 1945 at age seventy-five. Smith College honored her memory in 1967 with an exhibition and symposium on Crete.

TO FIND OUT MORE . . .

- Allsebrook, Mary Nesbit. *Born to Rebel: the Life of Harriet Boyd Hawes.* Oxford: Oxbow Books, 1992.

- Read, Phyllis J., and Bernard L. Witleib. *The Book of Women's Firsts.* New York: Random House, 1992.

- Sicherman, Barbara, and Carol Hurd Green, eds. *Notable American Women: The Modern Period. A Biographical Dictionary.* Cambridge, MA: The Belknap Press of Harvard University Press, 1980.

Elizabeth Lee Hazen, 1885–1975

In 1948, with chemist Rachel Brown, the microbiologist Elizabeth Lee Hazen discovered the first safe and effective fungicide, Nystatin. Its most important use was in combating fungal invaders like yeast infections in humans, but it also proved useful in fighting Dutch Elm disease, molds threatening damp works of art, and molds in cattle feed and other stored foods.

Elizabeth Hazen was born in rural Rich, Mississippi, to Baptist cotton farmers. Both parents died when Elizabeth was a toddler, and she and her sister were brought up by her uncle and his wife. Hazen earned a B.S. from the Mississippi Industrial Institute and College in 1910. She spent several years teaching science to Mississippi high schoolers during the school year and taking classes during the summer. She had saved most of her earnings for graduate school.

In 1916 Hazen was finally able to enroll at Columbia University. She quickly earned her master's degree, but further study was interrupted by World War I. She worked in Army diagnostic laboratories during and after the war. Columbia finally granted her a Ph.D. in microbiology in 1927; she was forty-two.

Hazen spent two decades establishing herself as an authority on the identification of fungi. She taught at Columbia and spent a good deal of time in the lab, at first studying a wide range of infectious diseases, then narrowing her interests to the field of mycology, or the study of fungi. At the Columbia University Mycology Laboratory, she began to look for a naturally occurring fungicide that might prove as useful against diseases caused by fungi as penicillin had against bacterial diseases.

A chemist, Rachel Brown, joined Hazen in her search. Hazen collected soil samples from many parts of the country, cultured any microorganizms that showed activity, and passed them on to Brown. The chemist prepared extracts from the cultures, testing them on preselected fungi. They literally hit pay dirt when, in 1948, a sample yielded two fungicides, actidone and a brand-new substance that the researchers named Nystatin for the New York State Department of Health.

The fungicide, which the two women patented in 1954, produced over $13 million for the Brown-Hazen Fund. Brown and Hazen refused to profit personally from their discovery, and instead set up a trust to fund research grants in their chosen fields. Hazen continued her rigorous schedule of research despite the ulcers that had plagued her throughout her career. She spent her last two years in the Seattle retirement home where her sister lived. She died in 1973.

> **Hazen discovered the first safe and effective fungicide.**

TO FIND OUT MORE ...

- Baldwin, Richard S. *The Fungus Fighters: Two Women Scientists and Their Discovery.* Ithaca, NY: Cornell University Press, 1981.

- O'Hern, Elizabeth Moot. *Profiles of Pioneer Women Scientists.* Washington, D.C.: Acropolis Books, Ltd., 1986.

- Sicherman, Barbara, and Carol Hurd Green, eds. *Notable American Women: The Modern Period. A Biographical Dictionary.* Cambridge, MA: The Belknap Press of Harvard University Press, 1980.

- Vare, Ethlie Ann, and Greg Ptacek. *Mothers of Invention: From the Bra to the Bomb, Forgotten Women and their Unforgettable Ideas.* New York: William Morrow and Company, Inc., 1988.

Leta Anna Stetter Hollingworth, 1886–1939

The educational psychologist Leta Stetter Hollingworth was a staunch feminist who used "masculine" scientific tools to argue for the equality of the sexes. Much of her work was in direct opposition to the prevailing trends in psychology, which tended to use those same tools to justify women's low status. Hollingworth's work helped to give the suffrage movement some of its scientific ammunition.

Margaret Stetter gave birth to her first child, Leta, in a dugout on a homestead in newly settled Chadron, Nebraska. Her father John was a cowboy and jack-of-all-trades who handed Leta and her siblings over to his parents-in-law when Margaret died after giving birth to their third baby girl in 1890. In 1898, when Leta was twelve, John Stetter remarried and moved the children to his home in Valentine, Nebraska. Leta's new stepmother, however, was antagonistic toward her, and her time in her father's home was unhappy.

At the University of Nebraska, Stetter aspired to be a writer, but prudently earned a teaching certificate as well. Despite high marks from literature and creative writing professors, she had to fall back on the certificate when she graduated in 1906. She taught until she was married, two years later, to Harry Levi Hollingworth, a college classmate. The couple moved to New York City, where Harry Hollingworth was studying psychology at Columbia University.

Marriage somewhat tied Leta Hollingworth's hands. Married women could not teach in New York public schools, and her writing still received little attention. She decided to go back to school, earning an M.A. in education and psychology in 1913 and a Ph.D. in 1916, both from Columbia. On her graduation, she took a position at Teachers College, where she would continue her research for the rest of her life.

At Columbia, Hollingworth had challenged the popular notion that women were physically and emotionally impaired by menstruation. She tested groups of women and men at all stages of the month for physical and mental functioning, and reported in her dissertation, *Functional Periodicity*, that she had found no differences between the sexes. She continued to pick apart such discriminatory ideas in her work at Teachers College, finding that the physical aspects of femininity—maternity and the menstrual cycle—were often used to justify discrimination against women.

Hollingworth's work focused on the development of gifted children.

Hollingworth began to focus on child psychology in the 1920s and 1930s. She centered her energies on unusually bright children, and in 1936 became the director of a special school for gifted children, the Speyer School. She published some of her observations in her influential *Children Above 180 I.Q.* (published posthumously in 1942). She came to the conclusion that the best I.Q. range for total adjustment was between 125 and 155 points. Her work with her gifted students had impressed her with the loneliness of children with exceptionally high intelligence.

In 1938, both Hollingworths were awarded honorary degrees from their undergraduate alma mater, the University of Nebraska. Leta Hollingworth died the next year at fifty-three years old. In 1940 Teachers College remembered her with a conference in her honor on the education of gifted children.

TO FIND OUT MORE . . .

- Haber, Louis. *Women Pioneers of Science.* New York: Harcourt Brace Jovanovich, 1979.

    - Hollingworth, Harry L. *Leta Stetter Hollingworth: A Biography.* Bolton, MA: Anker, 1990.

    - O'Connell, Agnes N., and Nancy Felipe Russo. *Models of Achievement: Reflections of Eminent Women in Psychology.* New York: Columbia University Press, 1983.

- Sicherman, Barbara, and Carol Hurd Green, eds. *Notable American Women: The Modern Period. A Biographical Dictionary.* Cambridge, MA: The Belknap Press of Harvard University Press, 1980.

Karen Danielsen Horney, 1885–1952

. . . .

Karen Horney was one of the earliest feminist psychiatrists and psychoanalysts. The German-born Horney took issue with certain aspects of Freudian theory, especially his more condescending concepts, like the idea that women suffer from "penis envy." In fact, she suggested that women had the more fulfilling role in childbearing and rearing, and that, if anything, it was men who suffered from an inferiority complex because they lacked wombs.

Horney was born in Blankenese, Germany, near Hamburg. Her Dutch/Norwegian parents separated when she was young, causing the girl much trauma. She ended up identifying with her mother's independent point of view; Clotilde Danielsen chafed under her older, more traditional husband's expectations of her. Later, when Karen married a man much like her father who opposed her plans to continue her education, her mother was very supportive.

An intensely interested student, Karen married another student, Oskar Horney, while still studying medicine. Their three daughters were born while she worked for her doctorate, writing a thesis on "Post-Traumatic Psychoses" (1915). She also became interested in psychoanalysis, undergoing sporadic treatment herself for unresolved feelings about her parents, her own roles in her family and her career, and, increasingly, her marital difficulties. Financial troubles for Oskar Horney's investment firm in 1923 triggered disturbing changes in his personality. The couple separated in 1926.

During the twenties and thirties, Horney took on Freud's theories. She rejected out of hand the idea that female sexual development could be analyzed as an impoverished version of the male's. She saw the structure of Freud's argument as based on an assumption of women's inferior status. Her own experiences with her husband led her to publish a number of papers on the relationship between the sexes.

Horney found Berlin professionally stifling—she felt she could not speak her mind there. She also worried increasingly about growing bias against her field as a "Jewish science." In 1932 she took advantage of an opportunity to move to the United States offered her by Franz Alexander, an old Berlin colleague. With her seventeen-year-old daughter Renate, she moved to Chicago to become the assistant director of the Chicago Institute of Psychoanalysis. Once she arrived, however, Horney found that her old colleague (the Institute's director) considered her differences with Freudian theory too radical, and she left only two years later for New York City.

She established a successful practice as a psychoanalyst in the city and taught at the New York Psychoanalytic Institute and the New School for Social Research. She continued to criticize Freudian theory, publishing a book on the subject (*New Ways in Psychoanalysis*) in 1939. Again her ideas were considered too radical, and when more conservative forces at the Institute blocked her training privileges there, she resigned in protest.

There were other psychoanalysts who felt much as Horney did about the restrictions within the field. In 1941, together with Erich Fromm, Clara Thompson, and Harry Stack Sullivan, Horney founded the Association for the Advancement of Psychoanalysis for the newer, more radical breed. The new Association spawned a school, the American Institute for Psychoanalysis, and a journal, the *American Journal of Psychoanalysis*. Until her death in 1952, Horney worked as dean of the Institute and editor of the *Journal*.

Horney's assault on many of Freud's most fundamental ideas raised eyebrows.

TO FIND OUT MORE . . .

- Quinn, Susan. *A Mind of Her Own: The Life of Karen Horney.* New York: Summit Books, 1987.
- Rubins, Jack L. *Karen Horney: Gentle Rebel of Psychoanalysis.* New York: Dial Press, 1978.
- Sayers, Janet. *Mothers of Psychoanalysis.* New York: W.W. Norton, 1991.
- Sicherman, Barbara, and Carol Hurd Green, eds. *Notable American Women: The Modern Period. A Biographical Dictionary.* Cambridge, MA: The Belknap Press of Harvard University Press, 1980.

Ida Henrietta Hyde, 1857–1945

It took Ida Hyde a long time to earn her doctorate in physiology. Hindered by low finances and resistance to women in science, she spent twenty-three years working to complete her combined high school, college, and graduate education. Near the end of her distinguished career in physiology, she gave generously to fund scholarships and a fellowship for young women in the sciences.

Ida Hyde's parents emigrated from Württemburg, Germany, to the United States, where they changed their name from Heidenheimer to Hyde. Ida, one of four children, was born in Davenport, Iowa. At sixteen she was apprenticed to a millinery business in Chicago. Determined to educate herself, she managed to divide her time between work and the Chicago Athenaeum, a school for working students. At twenty-four she left her job for her first year of college at the University of Chicago.

Her money ran out after only a year, however, and Hyde was forced to find a job teaching in the Chicago public schools, where she stayed for the next seven years. Finally she was able to return to college at Cornell University, where she earned a bachelor's degree in 1891. She enrolled at Bryn Mawr College, where she studied under Thomas Hunt Morgan (Nobel Prize in Physiology or Medicine, 1993) and physiologist Jacques Loeb. In 1893 she was invited to conduct research at Strassburg University in Germany.

Funded by the Association of Collegiate Alumnae (later the American Association of University Women), Hyde took the offer. She ran into institutional resistance there, however—the University turned down her petition to take her Ph.D. examination—and transferred to Heidelberg.

Hyde had hoped to work with a distinguished Heidelberg physiologist, Wilhem Kühne, but found him extremely prejudiced against women. Other faculty members, however, took her side, and in 1896 she was awarded her doctorate. She graduated with high but not the highest honors, since Kühne opposed the university's highest academic degree being given to a woman. She was the first woman to earn an academic (as opposed to an honorary) Ph.D. at Heidelberg.

She spent some time before her return to America that fall working at the Heidelberg Table of the Zoological Station in Naples. Back in America she worked to establish an organization to help other women conduct research in Naples, the Naples Table Association for Promoting Scientific Research by Women. In 1898 Hyde was hired by the University of Kansas as an associate professor of physiology, and in 1905 she was promoted to full professor.

Hyde's scientific work was quite broad within her field; she was interested in both invertebrates and vertebrates. Late in her career she investigated the effects of radium on organisms. She was recognized for her work in 1902, when she became the first woman elected to membership in the American Physiological Association (and the only one for the next dozen years).

> *Opposition from the man she had hoped to study under kept Hyde from earning highest honors with her doctorate.*

Hyde continued her patronage of women, founding scholarships at both Cornell and the University of Kansas. She also gave $25,000 to establish a fellowship in her name with the American Association of University Women, the same organization that had made possible her study in Germany. After two and a half decades of research and teaching, Hyde retired to California. She died at age eighty-eight in Berkeley, California.

TO FIND OUT MORE . . .

- *The National Cyclopedia of American Biography* B, pp. 146–47. New York: J.T. White.

- Ogilvie, Marilyn Bailey. *Women in Science.* Cambridge, MA: The MIT Press, 1986.

- Sicherman, Barbara, and Carol Hurd Green, eds. *Notable American Women: The Modern Period. A Biographical Dictionary.* Cambridge, MA: The Belknap Press of Harvard University Press, 1980.

Libbie Henrietta Hyman, 1888–1969

Zoologist Libbie Henrietta Hyman was something of a maverick in her personal life, a loner whose colleagues sometimes found her abrasive. Her devotion to her field focused on a similarly unpopular group—the boneless invertebrates. She quickly became the leading expert on lower invertebrates, which were largely unexplored when, between 1916 and 1967, she did her extensive research.

Hyman's childhood was a difficult one. Her parents were often at odds with each other; the immigrant family was beset by financial troubles, and her mother was an unpleasantly dominating force in Libbie's life. To escape, she developed an interest in the flora of her Fort Dodge, Iowa, home. She also became a fiercely precocious student, graduating early as valedictorian of her 1905 high school class. She lived at home until she was forty-one, when her critical mother died.

After a few years' work pasting labels in a Mother's Rolled Oats factory and study-

ing science on her own time, Hyman was offered a scholarship in 1906 to the University of Chicago. She had intended to study botany, but felt that the department was anti-Semitic; she switched to zoology. Her mentor in the department, Charles Manning Child, directed her doctoral work after she earned her B.S. in 1910. She did some postdoctoral teaching in the department after she received her Ph.D. in 1915, and began to publish articles and laboratory manuals.

Soon after her mother died, she moved to New York City to work at the American Museum of Natural History, where colleagues considered her an odd bird and gossiped about her cigar smoking habits (a fabrication). Her avid interest in the unexplored lower invertebrates quickly established her as an authority; colleagues often sent her odd specimens to identify. She so enjoyed the taxonomy of her homely group that she began to compile a comprehensive reference series on the biology of invertebrates. The six-volume work, *The Inverte-brates*, took nearly thirty years to put to-gether and was published between 1940 and 1967. Hailed as a work of astounding depth and breadth, it has become a classic.

In 1966, Parkinson's disease, which had plagued her since age seventy-one, forced Hyman to give up her pursuit of two more volumes for her definitive series, one on arthropods and another on the higher mollusks. She con-tinued to work at the American Museum of American History un-til her death in 1969.

> *Her massive work*
> **The Invertebrates**
> *still stands as a*
> *classic.*

TO FIND OUT MORE . . .

- Riser, Nathan W., and M. Patricia Morse, eds. *MBiology of the Turbellaria*. New York: McGraw–Hill, 1974.

- Sicherman, Barbara, and Carol Hurd Green, eds. *Notable American Women: The Modern Period. A Biographical Dictionary*. Cambridge, MA: The Belknap Press of Harvard University Press, 1980.

- Yost, Edna. *American Women of Science*. New York: J.B. Lippincott Company, 1955.

Sara Claudia Murray Jordan, 1884–1959

The gastroenterologist Sara Jordan believed in prevention as the most important part of medical treatment. This is not surprising, considering that her specialty was treating ulcer-prone Boston businessmen. She counseled them to reduce stress in the simplest possible ways. "Every businessman over fifty should have a daily nap and a nip," she once said, "a short nap after lunch, and a relaxing highball before dinner." Although ulcers are now treated more effectively with antibiotics, Jordan's advice was the best then available and brought comfort to many.

Patrick Andrew Murray, from County Cork, Ireland, had seven children with his wife Maria in Newton, Massachusetts. His carriage and auto body repair shop supported the large family. Sara Murray, the second eldest, aspired as a child to become a doctor. Her father opposed her plan early on, but when it later became clear that she had made up her mind, her family supported her in her choice.

Sara Murray was an accomplished scholar. She went from the Newton public schools to Radcliffe where she earned her A.B. in classics in only three years. From Radcliffe, she went to the University of Munich to study for a Ph.D. in archaeology and classical philology, which she earned after four years of study in 1908. In 1913, she married Sebastian Jordan, a German lawyer from her University of Munich days. The marriage was not a happy one. The Jordans had a daughter, Mary Stuart, in 1914, but World War I divided the couple, and Mary went home to her parents with her five-month-old daughter. The Jordans' divorce was finalized in 1921.

Jordan eventually moved with Mary into her own home in Brookline. During her medical school years, however (1917–1921), her parents were helpful and encouraging. Medical school presented problems that her other academic work had not; Tufts College kept her on "probationary" status after she had completed all her premed courses. She had to threaten to go to the AMA in order to be recognized as a student eligible for an M.D. In 1921 she graduated at the top of her class.

An internship at the Worcester Memorial Hospital and training in gastroenterology in Chicago gave Jordan the background necessary to become part of an unusual arrangement. In 1922 she established a group practice with two surgeons and an anesthesiologist. The Lahey Clinic, named for one of its surgeons, was one of very few independent clinics at the time—most Boston medicine was linked to three major medical schools. The clinic was highly successful, and Jordan's expertise was a major factor.

Jordan's expertise was a major factor in the early success of the Lahey Clinic.

She stressed noninvasive treatment for her mostly wealthy, high-strung gastrointestinal patients. She treated them with good humor and strict advice whenever possible, outlining a program of enforced rest and regulated diet. Her popularity and erudition led to a side career in writing. She published a cookbook in 1951, *Good Food for Bad Stomachs*. After her retirement in 1958, she also wrote a syndicated column, "Health and Happiness." Her simple, commonsense approach and scholarly background made her writing both interesting and sensible.

Jordan was honored by her colleagues with appointments to the presidency of the American Gastroenterology Association and to the board of trustees of Tufts University. In retirement, she followed her own advice, enjoying plenty of recreational time playing golf and seeing her five grandchildren. She diagnosed her own colon cancer, which took her life at the age of seventy-five.

TO FIND OUT MORE . . .

- Read, Phyllis J. and Bernard L. Witleib. *The Book of Women's Firsts.* New York: Random House, 1992.

- Sicherman, Barbara, and Carol Hurd Green, eds. *Notable American Women: The Modern Period. A Biographical Dictionary.* Cambridge, MA: The Belknap Press of Harvard University Press, 1980.

- *Sara Murray Jordan: A Memorial Volume.* Cambridge, MA: Harvard University Print. Office, 1994.

- Jordan's papers are at the Schlesinger Library at Radcliffe College.

Helen Dean King, 1869–1955

. . . .

elen Dean King, biologist, caught the attention of the national press with her studies on the breeding of rats. Her work was of great importance to her field—she successfully domesticated the Norway rat for research purposes, for example—but the press focused on the sensationalistic aspects of her work. When she published her findings on the benefits of inbreeding in laboratory rat strains, a headline exaggerated wildly: "Dr. King Quizzed on Kin Marriage Theory: Home Folk Shocked by Advocacy of Human Inbreeding." Death threats followed.

King was born in Oswego, New York. Both parents came from comfortable families who owned leather companies, and Helen's childhood was financially secure. She attended her father's alma mater, the Owego Free Academy, before attending Vassar from 1888 to 1892. She went from Vassar to Bryn Mawr College to pursue a doctorate, studying morphology, paleontology, and physiology.

An early scientific influence was Thomas Hunt Morgan, her morphology professor. Morgan has been called the "father of modern genetics"; he proved the existence of genes. She stayed at Bryn Mawr as an assistant for five years after she earned her Ph.D. there in 1899. In 1906 a position as an assistant in anatomy at the University of Pennsylvania became available, and it was only a short move from Penn to Philadelphia's Wistar Institute of Anatomy and Biology, where she would stay for forty-one years (1908–1949).

King's research at the Wistar Institute with Norway and albino rats proved shocking to many. The fact that a woman worked with rats in the first place was problematic. One reporter gushed about his "wonder" at "the spectacle of a woman holding a rat in the palm of her hand." The same reporter found it surprising that "one of the greatest authorities on rats in the country is a very human and thoroughly feminine woman."

Her conclusions, however, drew the nastiest attention.

Helen King studied twenty-five generations of albino rats to examine the effects of inbreeding. When she published her findings that brother-sister matings produced large, healthy rats, exaggeration abounded. The press claimed that King thought incest taboos kept humanity from naturally improving itself through consanguineous marriage, and King had to suffer a deluge of disapproval.

From 1919 to 1949 King worked to develop domesticated strains of the Norway rat. The rat, which was considered too wild to breed in a laboratory, produced an amazing array of types under King's care, including curly-haired rats and chocolate-colored rats. More importantly for biology, she bred rats with specific genetic characteristics that were tailor-made for specific research projects, as well as a stable, pure strain that became a laboratory standard.

Helen King retired at age eighty. She lived in Philadelphia for the six years before her death in 1955.

Her controversial findings on inbreeding in rats caused a furor in the press.

TO FIND OUT MORE ...

- Ogilvie, Marilyn Bailey. *Women in Science*. Cambridge, MA: The MIT Press, 1986.

Flemmie Kittrell, 1904–1980

H ome economics is a field that con-
jures up images of young women
learning to bake the perfect pot roast for
their future husbands. Women like Flemmie
Kittrell made it mean much more. She
served as the head of the home economics
department at Howard University for nearly
thirty years, using her position to conduct
studies of nutrition problems in Liberia and
India. She set up programs to train women
in nutrition and child care in India and in
Zaire, contributing immensely to the general welfare.

Flemmie Kittrell was the third youngest
of nine children born to James Lee Kittrell
and Alice Mills Kittrell in Henderson, North
Carolina. Both parents were the offspring of
Cherokee and African-American parents.
Their home was warm and supportive for
Flemmie, the youngest daughter, and she
proved a quick learner in the North Carolina
public schools.

She enrolled at Hampton Institute (later
renamed Hampton University) and was
much encouraged by her professors to consider graduate school. She was initially hesi-

tant—graduate school was not considered an
option for African-American women when
she graduated in 1928. Still, the enthusiastic
support of her family and professors bol-
stered her courage, and after a year spent
teaching at Bennett College in Greensboro,
she applied to Cornell University. She was
accepted, and went on to earn an M.A. in
1930 and a Ph.D. with honors in 1938.

After graduating from Cornell, Kittrell
returned to Bennett to teach, then moved
to her alma mater, Hampton Institute, to direct its home economics division and serve
as dean of women. In 1944 she landed a position as the head of the Home Economics
Department at Howard University. She
spent most of her professional life there,
working to make her field fit a more scientifically grounded model.

Kittrell thought that home economics,
like any other science, should be based on
research. She began to apply that theory in
a 1947 study of nutrition in Liberia. She
found that 90 percent of the population suffered from "hidden hunger," or inadequate
nutrition, because their diet consisted

mostly of rice and cassava. She proposed several remedies to the Liberian government, suggesting that the fishing industry should be enlarged, the agricultural industry improved, and the agricultural administration developed.

In 1950, assisted by a Fulbright program, she went to India to help Baroda University get its Home Economics college and nutritional research program under way. She returned in 1953 to work for the Agency for International Development, giving seminars and demonstrations. In 1952 she helped to establish the Congo Polytechnic Institute's School of Home Economics in Zaire. In 1957 she traveled to Japan, Hawaii, and West Africa; in 1959 to West and Central Africa; and in 1961 to Guinea. She occasionally encountered some resistance in cultures where women's education was not approved, but persistence paid off.

Kittrell also broke new ground at Howard University. She pushed for fifteen years for new facilities for her field, and the university's School of Human Ecology was dedicated in 1963. Kittrell retired at age seventy-three in 1972, although she continued to lecture and travel until two years before her death in 1980.

Her 1947 study of nutrition in Liberia found that 90 percent of the population suffered from "hidden hunger."

TO FIND OUT MORE . . .

- Smith, Jessie Carey. *Notable Black American Women.* Detroit, MI: Gale Research Inc., 1992.

- *Who's Who of American Women.* 12th Ed. Chicago: Marquis, 1982.

- Flemmie Kittrell's papers are in the archives at Hampton University and Howard University, and the Schlesinger Library at Radcliffe College has a transcript of her interview for the Black Women Oral History Project.

Sophia Josephine Kleegman, 1901-1971

· ·

Sophia Josephine Kleegman was one of the first gynecologists fully to incorporate the psychological issues associated with fertility into her medical practice. By confronting issues like performance anxiety, repression, and stress, she worked to change prevailing attitudes and to set her patients at ease.

Sophia Kleegman spent her first five years in Kiev, Russia. Her parents had four boys (all four died in childhood) and four girls, of whom Sophia was the youngest. The two eldest moved to the teeming immigrant neighborhood on the Lower East Side of New York City, where they worked in garment district sweatshops to earn the fare for their family's passage. The Kleegmans immigrated when Sophia was five, although she did not become a naturalized American citizen until she was seventeen.

While her parents and older sisters worked to support the family, Sophia and her younger sister Anna were encouraged

to pursue a profession. Sophia followed the same career path as Anna, graduating from the University and Bellevue Hospital Medical College (renamed the New York University College of Medicine) in 1924. Like Anna she chose gynecology and obstetrics, and in 1929 became New York University's first woman faculty member in obstetrics and gynecology at the College of Medicine.

In 1932 she married orthodontist John H. Sillman, but kept her own name. When they had their first child, Frederick, in 1937, Kleegman found that emergency obstetrical calls were too invasive for her to take, and so dropped that side of her practice. With hired help she was able to continue her work in gynecology while her two children were small.

Around the time of her marriage, Kleegman began her studies on fertility and conception. She was a sensitive physician who gently explored the psychological issues of performance and blame in conception. She took a straightforward approach to all aspects of conception, including controversial topics like birth control and artificial insemination. Indeed, she was one of the few physicians then willing to confront the psychological aspects of gynecological practice directly.

She was an early, outspoken advocate of the right to birth control. She toured widely to lecture on sex education and served for twenty-five years as the medical director of the New York State Planned Parenthood Association (1936–1961). At New York University, she argued for—and got—sex education included in the curriculum.

> Kleegman was an early and outspoken advocate of birth control.

Kleegman was as able in the laboratory as she was with patients and students. Her best-remembered contribution was her work with the "Pap smear" test developed by George Papanicolau; she further developed the test to yield more diagnostic information. Her candid style made her a popular lecturer at NYU, and she was an able administrator as well. The university made her its first female head of the NYU Medical Alumni Association in 1965.

Sophia Kleegman maintained her active, multifaceted schedule up until her death in New York City at the age of seventy. Her memory was honored by friends and peers at NYU by a professorship in human reproduction established in her name.

TO FIND OUT MORE . . .

- Obituary. *The New York Times,* Sept. 27, 1971.
- Sicherman, Barbara, and Carol Hurd Green, eds. *Notable American Women: The Modern Period. A Biographical Dictionary.* Cambridge, MA: The Belknap Press of Harvard University Press, 1980.
- Singer, Joy Daniels. *My Mother, The Doctor.* New York: Dutton, 1970.
- Kleegman's papers are at the Schlesinger Library at Radcliffe College.

Rebecca Craighill Lancefield, 1895–1981

Microbiologist Rebecca Lancefield was one of the researchers who contributed to the search for ways to fight streptococci, the group of bacteria that cause scarlet fever, erysipelas, and rheumatic fever, among other diseases. The International Congress of Microbiology sanctioned her method of identifying different types of streptococci, which appear confusingly similar under a microscope.

Rebecca Craighill was the child of an Army officer, and like any Army brat she spent her childhood in a series of homes that changed whenever her father was sent to a new post. She was born at Fort Wadsworth on Staten Island, New York, and her early education was a patchwork of public and private schools and private tutors. When she enrolled at Wellesley in 1912, she expected to study French and English, but soon became interested in zoology. She focused on bacteriology and spent some time catching up on chemistry.

On her graduation in 1916, Craighill was hired to teach mathematics and some unspecified science at a boarding school in Burlington, Vermont. When she arrived, it turned out that the science course she was to teach was geography. After saving almost half of her salary for graduate school, she won a scholarship for daughters of the military to enroll at Columbia University.

The catch was that she had to go to Teachers' College at Columbia, which then had no bacteriology or genetics courses that she wanted to take. She solved the problem by matriculating at Teachers' College but taking classes at the University's medical school. In 1918, after a year of productive work, she earned an M.A. through Teachers' College and married a student from her genetics course, Donald Lancefield.

For a few years, Rebecca Lancefield's career took a back seat to her husband's. She worked at Rockefeller Hospital while he earned his Ph.D., and taught briefly at the

University of Oregon when he had a position there. But in 1922 the couple returned permanently to New York, where Rebecca began her lifelong work on streptococci at the Rockefeller Institute and finished her Ph.D. at Columbia in 1925.

Her doctoral work was plagued by bad luck; she tried to develop an orderly system of classification for a particularly quirky strain of streptococcus. Still, her findings were later published in the *Journal of Experimental Medicine* (vol. 42). She persisted in investigating other strains of streptococci, and by the late twenties was making significant headway.

Lancefield isolated substances from her samples of streptococci that she found could be used to group them in five different types. She collaborated with other researchers abroad who were on the same track, and by 1940 she had emerged as a leader in the field. Her findings were the basis of the method of classification of streptococci adopted by the International Congress of Microbiology around 1940, and in 1943 she was elected president of the Society of American Bacteriologists.

She continued to clarify further the distinctions between different strains of strep-

> *Lancefield's work in microbiology spanned five decades and produced a new system of classification for streptococci.*

tococci, and was often consulted as an authority on the bacteria. In 1960 she used a dried sample from her 1935 work to identify a strain that was attacking lab mice. That same year, at age sixty-five, she was elected the first woman president of the American Association of Immunologists. And in 1970 she was the eleventh woman elected to the National Academy of Sciences.

Lancefield was active right up to her eighties, fielding other researchers' requests for advice on streptococci, conducting her own research and publishing her findings. She died in 1981 at age eighty-six.

TO FIND OUT MORE . . .

- O'Hern, Elizabeth Moot. *Profiles of Pioneer Women Scientists*. New York: Acropolis Books, 1985.
- Wannamaker, Lewis W. "Obituary: Rebecca Craighill Lancefield." *ASM News* 47 (1981): 555–9.

Amelia Rudolph Laskey, 1885-1973

Amelia Laskey was an uneducated Nashville housewife when she started watching birds. With no training and no immediate scientific network, she turned a hobby into a serious vocation, producing important studies on mockingbird and cowbird behavior. Although she was two years Laskey's junior, **Margaret Morse Nice** became her mentor through letters, encouraging her to publish her excellent articles.

Amelia Rudolph was the child of German immigrants Susan and Frank Rudolph. She was born in Bloomington, Indiana, and raised in Chicago, where she attended high school and secretarial classes and worked for the Oliver Typewriter Company as a stenographer until she married Frederick C. Laskey at the age of twenty-six. Ten years later, in 1921, the couple moved to Nashville, Tennessee.

Amelia Laskey was happy with her house outside Nashville. She created a wild garden in her four acres of back yard, and

dubbed the residence Blossomdell. She was an obsessively meticulous caretaker, and spent considerable effort in regularly cleaning the house and maintaining the grounds. In 1928 she went to her first meeting of the Tennessee Ornithological Society, and was immediately hooked. In 1930 she began her forty-two-year freelance writing career with a little article entitled "Attracting Birds to the Home" for the Tennessee Ornithological Society's journal, *The Migrant*.

Bird banding became a major interest for her. She obtained a banding license and began her long-range life studies of several species. A chimney swift she banded in 1940 showed up in Peru, revealing for the first time the swift's winter destination. She caught several species rare to Tennessee, including a Gambel's sparrow, which had never before been recorded in the state. She was also able to observe closely the mating habits of cowbirds, identifying new types of sexually aggressive behavior in which cowbirds of both sexes jealously placed themselves between their mates and possible rivals.

Laskey befriended neighborhood children, who knew her as "the lady who fixes birds." They brought her abandoned baby birds or sick ones she sometimes nursed back to health. One of these proved useful in her studies. She raised "Honey Child," a mockingbird, from a nestling. He lived with her for over fifteen years, providing an invaluable model for close study of mockingbird behavior. From Honey Child, Laskey learned that mockingbirds, unlike songbirds, do not inherit their songs. Honey Child learned and imitated the songs of the other feathered visitors to Laskey's home.

This amateur Nashville birdwatcher turned her hobby into a forty-two-year career—and was elected a fellow of the American Ornithologists' Union.

Laskey was as meticulous about her research as she was about her home. She set up hundreds of nesting boxes over her career in a huge park, in which she was able to observe the nesting habits of bluebirds. Maintaining the boxes, which were often the victims of vandals and careless groundskeepers, was a huge amount of work and Laskey wearied under the combined strain of ornithology and housework. Her friend Margaret Morse Nice pressed her to ease up on the housework, but Laskey continued to knock herself out doing everything just so.

The American Ornithologists' Union recognized her contributions in 1966 by electing her a fellow. She died seven years later at the age of eighty-eight.

TO FIND OUT MORE . . .

- Bonta, Margaret Meyers. *Women in the Field: America's Pioneering Naturalists.* College Station, TX: Texas A&M University Press, 1991.

- Goodpasture, Katharine A. "In Memoriam: Amelia Rudolph Laskey." *Auk* 92 (1975): 252–59.

Henrietta Swan Leavitt, 1868–1921

H enrietta Leavitt was nearly deaf. She never let the handicap block her in school or in work, and her scientific field—astronomy—benefited enormously from her diligent analysis of the skies. She methodically recorded her observations of the luminosity of thousands of stars, laying the groundwork for other researcher's flashier discoveries, and in the course of her career made a few important discoveries of her own.

Leavitt's conscientious and self-effacing nature was rooted in her childhood. Born in Lancaster, Massachusetts, one of seven children of a Congregationalist minister, she was raised in Cambridge, Massachusetts, until she was seven, when her family moved to Cleveland, Ohio. Originally interested in music, Leavitt attended Oberlin for two years before switching to Radcliffe College, then called the Society for Collegiate Instruction of Women.

Leavitt began working as a volunteer at the Harvard College Observatory in 1895, and was made a member of the permanent staff there in 1902. The director of the Observatory, Edward C. Pickering, appreciated Leavitt's quiet demeanor and hard work. In 1907 he handed over a major project to her.

The luminosity of stars had been carefully observed with the human eye for many years, and the Harvard Observatory had been recording these observations for the last three decades. Photographic plates, however, were not only a more objective method of recording luminosity, but they also proved able to pick up certain wavelengths that the human eye could not sense.

Using nearly three hundred plates, taken through thirteen different telescopes, Leavitt standardized such measurements with her analysis of a large group of stars near the Pole star, called the North Polar Sequence. In 1913, the International Committee on Photographic Magnitudes voted to adopt Leavitt's system as the standard for their Astrographic Map of the Sky, a huge project intended to catalog the positions of the stars.

Meanwhile, Leavitt's father had died and her mother had come to live with her in her Cambridge home. Her research continued undisturbed, and in her twenty-six years at the Observatory she made several important discoveries. Working with variable stars, stars that brighten and dim repeatedly, she established a relationship between the brightness of the star and the length of its period of pulsation. The longer the period, the brighter the star. The discovery made it possible for later researchers to measure the distance between such stars and the earth.

Leavitt also noted that redder stars were usually dimmer, sparking the line of inquiry that later, using much newer technology, distinguished between stars that gave off a red light and stars whose light turned red through the filter of particles between them and the Earth. She would undoubtedly have contributed far more had she not died early at the age of fifty-two.

> *The International Committee on Photographic Magnitudes voted to adopt Leavitt's system as the standard for their Astrographic Map of the Sky.*

TO FIND OUT MORE . . .

- *The National Cyclopaedia of American Biography XXV*, p. 163. New York: J.T. White.

- Ogilvie, Marilyn Bailey. *Women in Science*. Cambridge, MA: The MIT Press, 1986.

- Sicherman, Barbara, and Carol Hurd Green, eds. *Notable American Women: The Modern Period. A Biographical Dictionary*. Cambridge, MA: The Belknap Press of Harvard University Press, 1980.

Lena Levine, 1903–1965

The gynecologist and psychiatrist Lena Levine committed her considerable talents to the cause of legalized contraception. She worked for the Planned Parenthood Federation of America and for the International Planned Parenthood Federation. Her interests and influences were broad; she assisted with marriage counseling, abortion referrals, and group counseling on sex and contraception. Despite her radical work, however, she followed the lead of many other feminists of the time in *not* publicly supporting abortion, hoping to keep that sticky issue from complicating the fight for legalized birth control.

Lena was the baby in a family of seven children born to Sophie and Morris Levine, Russian Jewish emigrés who settled in Brooklyn. Her father, a clothing manufacturer, managed to support the family at a level somewhat above that of their mostly poor, mostly Jewish neighbors. Lena went to Girls High School in Brooklyn and to Hunter College, graduating with an A.B. in 1923. She then went on to medical school at Bellevue Hospital Medical College.

Two years after her graduation in 1927, she married a fellow student, Louis Ferber, but kept her own name. They moved to Brooklyn and did their residencies together at Brooklyn Jewish Hospital. When they finished, they set up a joint practice in their home, he as a general practitioner, she as a obstetrician and gynecologist. They had two children, Ellen Louise and Michael Allen. Michael barely survived an attack of viral encephalitis in early infancy; it left him with serious brain damage. After he turned six, he had to be put in an institution, where his mother visited him until her death.

Following hard on this tragedy was her husband's sudden death of a heart attack in 1943, a year after Michael's illness. Lena decided to give up obstetrics, a field that could take her away from her children at a moment's notice with a patient's call. She kept her practice in gynecology and began to study psychiatry. A Freudian, she opened another private practice in Manhattan, splitting her time between her gynecology patients in Brooklyn and the patients she counseled in Manhattan. When her daughter went off to college in 1957, she moved both her small practices to a new home in Greenwich Village.

All the time her children were growing up, Levine had been active in work for legalized birth control. She worked for Planned Parenthood (then called the Birth Control Federation of America), first in the American organization and later as the international organization's medical secretary. She worked as a marriage counselor at the Community Church of New York and organized group counseling programs on sexual problems and contraception. Her Special Consultation Bureau gave health advice and abortion referrals to pregnant women.

Levine's lectures and many publications aimed to wipe out many of the sexist myths associated with the physiology of "the emotional sex." She addressed adolescent sexuality, menopause, virginity, contraception, and sex in marriage in her many pamphlets, papers, and books on female sexuality. She lived in New York until her death at age sixty-one.

Levine was one of the early advocates for legalizing birth control in the U.S.

TO FIND OUT MORE . . .

- Gordon, Linda. *Woman's Body, Woman's Right: A Social History of Birth Control in America.* New York: Grossman, 1976.

- Sicherman, Barbara, and Carol Hurd Green, eds. *Notable American Women: The Modern Period. A Biographical Dictionary.* Cambridge, MA: The Belknap Press of Harvard University Press, 1980.

Esther Clayson Pohl Lovejoy, 1869–1967

Edward and Annie Clayson had their third of six children, Esther, in a logging camp near Seabeck, Washington. Edward was an unsuccessful jack-of-all-trades who worked briefly as a lumber merchant, a hotel manager, a farmer, and a newspaper editor without ever quite finding his niche. Esther's education was spotty; she attended a school at a lumber camp and took history lessons with a poor classics professor at a hotel her father managed. Despite this disadvantage, she decided on a career in medicine when she saw a woman doctor deliver her younger sister.

In 1890 Esther Clayson began work on her M.D. at the University of Oregon. She borrowed money and dropped out for a year to finance the degree, but still managed to complete the requirements in 1894 and win a medal for academic achievement. She was the school's first woman graduate to practice medicine. She married fellow student Emil Pohl immediately after gradu-

ation, and they opened a practice together in Portland.

In 1896 Esther's brothers convinced the young couple to move to Skagway, Alaska, where they became the first physicians in the area while Esther's brothers sold supplies to gold prospectors. The Pohls helped establish the Union Hospital there. Life was still rough in Alaska—the Pohls lived in a log cabin and used a dogsled to visit patients—but Emil Pohl fell in love with the territory and decided to stay. When Esther's brother Frederick was found murdered in 1899, she went home to Portland, but continued to visit Emil in the summers. Personal tragedy struck again in 1908, when their son died of septic peritonitis, and in 1911, when Emil Pohl died in Alaska of encephalitis.

Esther Pohl increased her political activity, becoming an active suffragist and prohibitionist. She married George Lovejoy, a businessman, in 1913, but divorced him only seven years later because he used her name to support causes she did not herself advocate. As a member of the American Medical Women's Association (AMWA), she agitated (unsuccessfully) for women physicians' right to serve in World War I, and followed through by volunteering as an American Red Cross nurse in Paris. In 1919 she published a book about her experiences there, *The House of the Good Neighbor.*

In 1918 Esther Lovejoy worked for the AMWA as a fundraiser for its war relief agency, the American Women's Hospitals Service(AWHS), giving lectures to groups of contributors on conditions in Europe. In 1919, she was made its director, a post she held for forty-eight years. After an unsuccessful bid for Congress in 1920, Lovejoy concentrated on her work for AWHS, working in Europe, writing her memoirs (*Certain Samaritans*), and lecturing to raise money. She was made president of the AMWA as well in 1932.

Her many honors and prizes included France's medal of the Legion of Honor, Greece's Gold Cross of the Order of George I, Yugoslavia's Gold Cross of Saint Sava, Jerusalem's Gold Cross of the Holy Sepulcher, and the AMWA's Elizabeth Blackwell Medal (twice). She resigned from her AWHS responsibilities at ninety-seven, five months before her death.

> *Lovejoy agitated (unsuccessfully) for women physicians' right to serve in World War I.*

TO FIND OUT MORE . . .

- Sicherman, Barbara, and Carol Hurd Green, eds. *Notable American Women: The Modern Period. A Biographical Dictionary.* Cambridge, MA: The Belknap Press of Harvard University Press, 1980.

- Lovejoy's papers are at the Schlesinger Library at Radcliffe College.

Lillien Jane Martin, 1851–1943

. . . .

Psychologist Lillien Martin was living proof that it is possible to start your life over from scratch. She did it twice. Martin didn't begin her career in science until she had already had a successful career in teaching and high school administration. She was forty-three and a vice principal at the San Francisco Girls' High School when she suddenly decided to return to school to become a psychiatrist. Twenty years later, she became the head of the psychiatry department at Stanford University—the first woman to head a department there. After her retirement, she tackled yet another career as a consulting psychologist, working with young children and the elderly.

Lillien, called Lillie Jane by her family, was the first of four children. Her father, a merchant, left his wife to raise the children alone when Lillie Jane was quite small, and it was her mother's determination to educate her children that led Lillien into teaching.

By sixteen she was teaching at an Episcopal girls' school in Racine, Wisconsin, near the college where her mother worked as a matron. She saved enough money from this job and another teaching position in Omaha, Nebraska, to pay her way when Vassar College accepted her as a freshman in 1876.

After her graduation from Vassar in 1880, Martin taught physics and chemistry in Indiana and San Francisco for fourteen years. In 1894 she resigned to go to the University of Göttingen, where she earned her Ph.D. in psychology in 1898. Her education in Europe made her part of the international psychological community; she returned often to Germany during her summers to study and published most of her work in German.

In 1899 she was hired by Stanford University as an assistant professor of psychology. Her teaching and administrative experience were helpful to her there, and she was steadily promoted to associate professor (1909), full professor (1911), and finally, at age sixty-four, department head (1915). Unfortunately she had to retire the next year at the age of sixty-five.

Retirement was certainly premature for Martin, and soon she had launched her third career as a psychologist. She founded mental heath clinics at the Mount Zion and Polyclinic Hospitals in San Francisco while running a successful private practice. In 1920 she established a pioneering program at Mount Zion for preschoolers. A run-in with a child's grandmother prompted her to explore gerontology, and by 1929 she had established an old age counseling center, supposed to be the country's first.

Constantly active and looking for ways to improve herself, she taught herself to drive in her seventies and then took a cross-country trip—alone—in a car. At seventy-eight she took a solo trip to Russia, and ten years later she took another trip alone to South America. She taught herself to touch-type when her hands were no longer steady enough to write neatly. She died at age ninety after twenty-five years of productive post-retirement work.

Martin's second career—begun at age forty-three—culminated in her appointment to the head of Stanford's psychology department.

TO FIND OUT MORE . . .

- DeFord, Miriam Allen. *Psychologist Unretired: The Life Pattern of Lillien J. Martin.* Stanford, CA: Stanford University Press, 1948.

- Ogilvie, Marilyn Bailey. *Women in Science.* Cambridge, MA: The MIT Press, 1986.

- Sicherman, Barbara, and Carol Hurd Green, eds. *Notable American Women: The Modern Period. A Biographical Dictionary.* Cambridge, MA: The Belknap Press of Harvard University Press, 1980.

Antonia Caetania Maury, 1866–1952

Antonia Maury was a brilliant and inventive astronomer who worked at the Harvard Observatory under Edward Pickering from 1887 to 1891. The fruit of her research at Harvard was a new, superior system for classifying stars. Mary's system turned out to play an important role in the development of theoretical astrophysics.

Maury's family, based in Cold Spring, New York, was deeply interested in science. Her uncle, Henry Draper, was an astronomer, and her father edited a geographical magazine. Antonia, the oldest child, attended Vassar College, earning a B.A. in 1887. Edward Pickering, the director of the Harvard College Observatory, was a family friend. On her graduation, Antonia's father asked Pickering if there might be a position for her at the Observatory. Pickering offered her a job at twenty-five cents an hour.

Edward Pickering was impressed with Maury's skill, but the job was frustrating for her. She found the routine numbing and

was dissatisfied with Pickering's system of classification. They soon clashed over her opinions, and her time at Harvard was not congenial. Her Uncle Henry Draper's widow, Mary, was the Observatory's main benefactor and sided with Pickering, advising him to treat her "as if she were a stranger, on a strictly business basis."

Despite the general unpleasantness, Maury forged ahead with her own work at the Observatory, coming up with a new system of classification that corrected Pickering's. She left Harvard in 1891 but returned regularly to make sure that the finished publication would have her name on it. In 1897 the finished catalog was published and began to attract interest and praise. Danish astronomer Ejnar Hertzsprung wrote Pickering to applaud Maury's catalog, which he regarded as a major advance. Pickering did not acknowledge Hertsprung's praise.

Maury returned to Harvard a year before Pickering's death in 1919 as a research associate. The new director, Harlow Shapley, was considerably more receptive to her ideas, and she was able to work for the Observatory on a project that had always intrigued her, spectroscopic binaries. These are stars that are distinguishable as binary stars (two stars rotating around one mass) on a spectrometer. Maury produced a classic study on them in 1933.

In 1935 she retired from Harvard to be the curator of her uncle's museum in Hastings-on-Hudson, New York. In 1943 the American Astronomical Society belatedly awarded her the Annie J. Cannon Prize for her 1897 system of classification. She died eight years later in Dobbs Ferry, New York.

> *Her clashes with Edward Pickering, director of Harvard's observatory, did not prevent her from publishing her groundbreaking astronomical catalog.*

TO FIND OUT MORE . . .

- Ogilvie, Marilyn Bailey. *Women in Science*. Cambridge, MA: The MIT Press, 1986.
- Maury's papers are at the Schlesinger Library at Radcliffe College.

Maria Gertrude Goeppert Mayer, 1906–1972

Physicist Maria Goeppert Meyer won a Nobel Prize in theoretical physics in 1963 for her theory of the structure of the atomic nucleus. This acknowledgment of her considerable achievements came near the end of a career in which she had been given little opportunity to prove herself. As the wife of a prominent scientist, she was unable to get a paying position in any university that hired him—nepotism rules forbade it. As a wife of a faculty member, however, she was allowed to work in university laboratories—for no pay and, often, no title. It was only in 1959, ten years after publishing her prizewinning theory, that she finally earned a post with her own title and pay.

Maria Gertrude Göppert (when she moved to the United States she changed her name to Goeppert) was the child of educators, raised in the German university town of Göttingen.

Mathematics, physics, and quantum mechanics were not closed to women in Germany in the twenties, but they were not the usual choices for young female university students. At Göttingen, Göppert excelled in all of them, propelled partly by her grief at her father's death in 1927 and her urge to become, like him, a university professor. Her mother began taking in boarders after her father's death. One of them was Joseph Edward Mayer, an American chemist who was visiting Göttingen on a Rockefeller grant to study with famed physicist James Franck. In 1930, he and Göppert were married.

That same year, she earned her Ph.D. with a dissertation that proved quite influential in her field, and again that same year, moved with her husband to the United States, where she became an American citizen. At Johns Hopkins, where her husband held a position, she did research (for no pay, under no title) in theoretical physical chemistry and had two children, Maria Anne (1933) and Peter (1938). At Columbia

University she worked under more or less the same conditions, this time in the S.A.M. Laboratory, participating in the Manhattan Project. In 1946, both Maria and Joseph Mayer were invited to join the faculty at the University of Chicago. There was a catch. She would finally be given the title of assistant professor, but no salary—not even when she became a full professor.

It was at Chicago that Goeppert Mayer began the work that led to her important discoveries. She became intrigued by patterns in the number of nuclear particles in stable elements. Struggling to find a way to explain the "magic numbers," she articulated a "shell theory" of electrons orbiting the nucleus. But her real breakthrough came when another Chicago researcher, Enrico Fermi, asked whether there were any indication of spin-orbit coupling. Mayer immediately solved the puzzle: The electrons spin as they circle the nucleus, like, she later explained, couples waltzing around a room.

Her paper on the theory was submitted to a journal in 1949. At the same time another researcher who had reached the same conclusions, Hans D. Jensen, submitted his to the same journal. They shared the Nobel

> *Goeppert Mayer did not win a paid research post until ten years after she published the theory that would eventually win her the Nobel Prize.*

with a third physicist, Eugene Wigner, fourteen years later. Ten years after publication, Goeppert Meyer was offered her first paid full professorship at the University of California in San Diego.

Sadly, she suffered a stroke only weeks after arriving in California. Although she was deaf in one ear and had almost completely lost the use of her left hand and arm, she continued to publish and do research. On being notified that she had won the Nobel, she exclaimed, "Good! I've always wanted to meet a king." She died of heart failure at the age of sixty-five.

TO FIND OUT MORE . . .

- Dash, Joan. *A Life of One's Own: Three Gifted Women and the Men They Married.* New York: Harper & Row, 1973.

- Opfell, Olga S. *The Lady Laureates: Women Who Have Won the Nobel Prize.* Metutchen, NJ: The Scarecrow Press, 1986.

- Read, Phyllis J. and Bernard L. Witleib. *The Book of Women's Firsts.* New York: Random House, 1992.

- Sicherman, Barbara, and Carol Hurd Green, eds. *Notable American Women: The Modern Period. A Biographical Dictionary.* Cambridge, MA: The Belknap Press of Harvard University Press, 1980.

Barbara McClintock, 1902-1992

Geneticist Barbara McClintock was the first American woman to win the Nobel prize in a scientific category by herself. Unlike **Gerty Cori**, who shared it with her husband Carl, and **Maria Goeppert Meyer**, who shared it with two other physicists, McClintock won the prize as a result of her solo work. It was an appropriate first for a woman who was known as a loner, as happiest in the company of her maize plants.

McClintock's parents actively discouraged their daughters from attending college, preferring that they get married. Barbara McClintock, however, spent her free time after graduation in the library. Her parents finally allowed her to enroll at Cornell University's College of Agriculture in 1919, where she majored in botany, a substitute for plant breeding, which was not open to female students.

McClintock stayed on after her graduation in 1923 to earn her Ph.D. in cytology, quickly gaining a reputation as a precocious young researcher. She became an instructor the year she earned her doctorate, 1927. Her work with Indian corn, or maize (*Zea mays*), was begun before she earned her degree.

This work ultimately led to her discovery of "jumping genes," which won her the Nobel Prize. In 1931, at the age of twenty-nine, she published "A Correlation of Cytological and Genetical Crossing-Over in *Zea Mays*" in *Proceedings of the National Academy*. Co-written with Harriet Creighton, the article was later hailed as a "cornerstone of modern genetics." McClintock and Creighton demonstrated that, as had been widely assumed, "Chromosomes exchange genetic information and physical material when they cross over early in meiosis." But, despite this impressive early accomplishment, McClintock's gender and idiosyncratic personality combined to bar her from academic advancement throughout her career.

McClintock was unable to win a faculty appointment at Cornell—in fact, no women were then on the Cornell Faculty. A brief stint in the late thirties at the University of Missouri was a bad experience. Peers and higher-ups saw only her eccentricities, not her brilliant, intuitive research. Once a school photographer snapped her scaling a wall to enter her accidentally locked office. A promotion seemed out of the question in light of her reputation for oddity. She finally found a permanent home at the Cold Spring Harbor genetics laboratory at the Carnegie Institution in Washington, D.C.

She presented the findings that eventually earned her the Nobel in 1951, but only a handful of geneticists even understood what she was talking about. Most thought that genes were fixed in place like links in a chain, but McClintock was proposing that some genes, called "dissociator" genes, "jump" about, moderating the effects of other, stationary genes. In 1956 she published her follow-up paper in the Cold Spring Harbor papers. Knowing that other researchers met her ideas with incredulity, McClintock did not try to publish the papers widely.

> Because she knew that other researchers viewed her ideas with incredulity, McClintock did not seek to publish them widely—but they eventually earned her a Nobel Prize.

Genetics caught up with her in the 1970s, when other researchers documented the same "jumping genes" in other plants and in fruit flies. Geneticists began to get excited about the idea, which some think will prove the key to solving the mysteries of previously incurable diseases like cancer.

In 1979 the prizes began to pour in, including a yearly $60,000 grant from the MacArthur Foundation.

In 1982 she met the news that she had won the Nobel—which she heard over the radio, since she had no telephone—with very little reaction. She took her customary walk in the woods before returning to comment that she had so enjoyed her intimate work with the maize plant that it seemed perhaps unfair to reward her for it. Nevertheless, the Nobel Committee heaped her work with long-overdue praise, ranking it with Crick and Watson's discovery of the double helix as "one of the two great discoveries of our time in genetics."

Barbara McClintock died ten years after receiving her prize. She was ninety years old.

TO FIND OUT MORE . . .

- Keller, Evelyn Fox. *A Feeling for the Organism: The Life and Work of Barbara McClintock.* San Francisco: W.H. Freeman, 1983.
- Opfell, Olga S. *The Lady Laureates: Women Who Have Won the Nobel Prize.* Metutchen, NJ: The Scarecrow Press, 1986.

Elizabeth McCoy, 1903-1978

Bacteriologist Elizabeth McCoy was a great contributor to her field in every way. She spent years searching for ways to use microorganisms in cleaning polluted water, valued her graduate students above her own academic accomplishments, and willed her family farms to her alma mater and longtime employer, the University of Wisconsin. She became a leader in an almost exclusively male scientific community, where her declaration that she never felt in any way that her gender was a problem for her colleagues is probably as much a testament to her as it is to them.

McCoy inherited her scientific curiosity from her mother, who, McCoy once mused, was "probably a frustrated medic." Esther Williamson reluctantly gave up the idea of attending medical school in Chicago and spent six years as an enthusiastic and active nurse, all the while postponing her marriage to Cassius McCoy. Elizabeth was raised on her father's farm in Madison, Wisconsin, where she showed such an intense interest in all farm matters that her father decided to train her to manage the farm instead of

her brother. She sped through high school, skipping fourth grade, and decided on a major in general bacteriology at the University of Wisconsin's College of Agriculture.

At Wisconsin, McCoy was just as precocious; she was hired as a research associate and enrolled in graduate classes for credit before she got her undergraduate degree. Her brilliant graduate work at Wisconsin on butyl alcohol-producing bacteria would eventually make her a leading authority on this group of organisms; in fact, it was she who proposed a name for the group, dubbing it *Clostridium acetobutylicum*. In 1930, the year after she earned her doctorate, Wisconsin hired her as an assistant professor of bacteriology. She would stay at Wisconsin for the rest of her career.

McCoy's interests branched out into several different areas of her field. She spent nearly thirty-five years researching the role of bacteria in lake ecosystems. Toward the end of her career, that knowledge made her an important contributor to the process of understanding the increasing problem of lake pollution. Her work with the clostridia led her, briefly, to Puerto Rico, where Wisconsin sent her to run a government project that established a butyl alcohol fermentation plant. The plant was plagued by a nasty outbreak of bacterial virus, or bacteriophage, that crippled the clostrida. Her inventive solution was to develop an altogether new culture of the bacteria, for which she would later receive a patent. She was an important contributor to the search for a usable type of *Penicillinum*; she found Strain X1612, which made penicillin usable for civilians. Other research included work on mastitis in dairy cattle, botulinum food poisoning, and bacteriophages.

> *McCoy showed such an intense interest in farm matters that her father trained her to manage the family farm.*

In every area of bacteriology she studied, she quickly emerged as a leader, despite the rarity of women in her field. She was devoted to her students, whom she called her "proudest endeavor." Her colleagues were lavish in their praise of her. One longtime co-worker of hers described her as "posessing an unusual combination of statesmanship and diplomacy . . . she has the cooperation of everyone with whom she works." She was active in her field even after she retired in 1973, and in fact died while still working vigorously on an effort to treat sewage with bacteria—a typically humanitarian project. She left her family farms, her lifelong home and joy, to Wisconsin.

TO FIND OUT MORE . . .

- O'Hern, Elizabeth Moot. *Profiles of Pioneer Women Scientists.* Washington, D.C.: Acropolis Books, Ltd., 1985.

- Sarles, W.B. "Obituary: Elizabeth McCoy." *ASM News* 44 (1978): 266–7.

Anita Newcomb McGee, 1864-1940

· ·

Physician Anita Newcomb McGee made use of her prominent social position in Washington, D.C., and her experience as a doctor to establish the Army Nurse Corps during the Spanish-American War at the turn of the century. For her work she was appointed Acting Assistant Surgeon General and given a rank commensurate with that of an army officer. When she died in 1940 at age seventy-five, she was buried in Arlington National Cemetery with full military honors.

Anita Newcomb was the first of three girls born to the intellectual Mary Caroline Newcomb and eminent astronomer Simon Newcomb. The family lived comfortably in Washington, D.C. When Newcomb was eighteen, she spent three years in Europe, where she received her undergraduate education at Cambridge University and the University of Geneva. She avoided offers of marriage, preferring to have her father's opinion on the matter.

Newcomb returned to Washington, D.C. in 1885. In 1888, she marred anthropologist and geologist William John McGee, like her father a self-made man and a scientist. They had a daughter, Cloth, the next year, but Anita Newcomb's studies and other activities took precedence over further children, and their son Eric was not born until 1902. In 1892, McGee earned her medical degree from Columbian University (later renamed George Washington University).

After studying gynecology at Johns Hopkins University, Newcomb practiced for a brief period. Soon, however, she gave up practicing medicine in favor of organizational activities, where she could better exert the considerable influence of her charismatic personality. She held leadership positions in the American Association for the Advancement of Science, the Women's Anthropological Society, and the Daughters of the American Revolution. It was under the auspices of the DAR and through her social connections that she proposed to organize a new Army-connected group of fully qualified nurses to serve during the Spanish-American War.

The organization was designed in part to compensate for the failings of the increasingly disorganized Red Cross. Unfortunately for Newcomb, criticisms of the Red Cross were unwelcome at the time, and she made enemies who shut down her Army career fairly quickly. Before her resignation, McGee drafted part of a bill that established the Army Nurse Corps. The final bill included an addition that stipulated that the director of the Corps must be a graduate nurse. As a physician, McGee was thus shut out of her position as director.

Nevertheless, her commitment to nurses was not dampened; she continued to work for and with them, heading the Society of Spanish-American War Nurses for six years. In 1905, she went with many of these nurses to Japan, where they served during the Russo-Japanese War. For this work and for her supervision of hospitals in Korea, Japan, and Manchuria, the Japanese government awarded her the Imperial Order of the Sacred Crown.

Newcomb lived out her later years de-

> *McGee worked to establish the Army Nurse Corps during the Spanish-American War.*

voted to her son. Tragically, he died in an accident at age twenty-eight. Anita McGee died ten years later in Washington, D.C. at the age of seventy-six.

TO FIND OUT MORE . . .

- *The National Cyclopedia of American Biography* X, p. 350. New York: J.T. White.

- Sicherman, Barbara, and Carol Hurd Green, eds. *Notable American Women: The Modern Period. A Biographical Dictionary.* Cambridge, MA: The Belknap Press of Harvard University Press, 1980.

- Obituary. *The Washington Post,* Oct. 6, 1940.

- McGee's papers are at the Library of Congress and in the National Archives.

Alice Woodby McKane, 1865-1948

. . . .

Alice McKane was half of a dynamic husband-wife team devoted to bettering the status of African-Americans. McKane and her husband, both physicians, organized health care facilities and training schools in the rural South and in Liberia. McKane also found time to write in her later years, publishing a book of her poems at age forty-nine.

Alice Woodby's childhood was full of loss. She was born in 1865 in Bridgewater, Pennsylvania, in 1865, and lost her parents, Charles Woodby and Elizabeth B. Frasier Woodby, before she was seven years old. She also lost her eyesight for a time, recovering after three years of blindness. She attended public schools until age twenty-one and the Institute for Colored Youth in Pennsylvania until age twenty-four. In 1889 she enrolled at the Women's Medical College of Pennsylvania.

Less than a year after she earned her medical degree in 1892, Alice Woodby married another practicing physician, Cornelius McKane. He was the grandson of a Liberian King who had been born in British Guiana; in time he became a great early civil rights activist in America. McKane was, variously, a clergyman, teacher, scholar, author, and speaker. Alice McKane was his match in drive and philanthropic leanings, and soon after their wedding she urged him to help her with a project she had in mind.

McKane wanted to open doors in medicine for other African-American women, and in 1893 the McKanes founded southeast Georgia's first training school for nurses. The first students graduated two years later, and in the meantime the McKanes and their trainees ran a much-needed clinic out of the school, treating local citizens for no fee. They were obliged to refuse about ten patients per week because of short resources, which were supplemented only by donations from local churches.

The couple traveled to Monrovia, Liberia, to work under similarly uncharted conditions. Alice McKane worked as a medical examiner for the United States government, overseeing the health of Civil War veterans living there. During her stay she co-organized and headed the department of women's diseases at Monrovia's fledgling hospital. Her work there soon threatened her health, however, and she returned with her husband to Savannah, Georgia, to recover from an African fever. By 1896, however, she was back on her feet.

Back in Georgia, the McKanes turned their project into the McKane Hospital for Women and Children and Training School for Nurses. Local white doctors helped with donations of their time and money. The McKanes, however, had three children around the time the hospital was founded, and after it was running they decided to leave Georgia in search of better education for them.

The family moved to Boston, where Alice McKane was a member of the NAACP and an active suffragist. She practiced medicine for many years, focusing on women's diseases. She also maintained her commitment to introducing other women to medicine, teaching nursing students at the Plymouth Hospital. She wrote in her spare time, publishing a book on healing, *The Fraternal Society Sick Book*, in 1913. A year later, her collection of poetry, *Clover Leaves*, was published.

Alice McKane died at age eighty-three.

With her husband Cornelius, McKane founded a training school for nurses and a free clinic in southeast Georgia.

TO FIND OUT MORE...

- Davis, Marianna W., ed. *Contributions of Black Women to America.* Vol. II. Columbia, SC: Kenday Press, 1982.

- Smith, Jessie Carey. *Notable Black American Women.* Detroit, MI: Gale Research Inc., 1992.

- *Who's Who in Colored America.* Vol. I. New York: Who's Who in Colored America Corp., 1927.

Aimee Semple McPherson, 1890–1944

A imee Semple McPherson, evangelist and faith healer, singlehandedly established a Pentecostal sect that in 1980 numbered nearly ninety thousand members. She was a figure of enormous charisma and flamboyance who appeared onstage dressed in white gown and shoes and a blue robe, leading revivals with a professional choir, an orchestra, and a brass band, while enthralled congregants spoke in tongues. Her religious empire at one time included a 500-watt radio station, a monthly magazine, and four hundred branch churches. Despite the commercialism of her work, she used her power for enormous good, establishing philanthropic services for her poorer congregants and a Bible college that graduated more than three thousand ordained missionaries.

Aimee Elizabeth Kennedy was born in Canada near Ingersoll, Ontario, where her father ran a farm and led the local Methodist choir. Her mother dedicated her, at six months of age, to God's work in a Salvation Army ceremony. At seventeen Aimee was converted in a Pentecostal revival by Robert James Semple, whom she married shortly thereafter. She was ordained a Pentecostal preacher the following year, and the couple traveled about, conducting revivals together.

In 1910, Aimee, pregnant, and Robert left for China to spread the Word. Unfortunately, Robert died, apparently of typhoid fever, soon after their arrival. After the birth of their baby, Roberta Star Semple, Aimee Semple returned to the United States to work with her mother for the Salvation Army in New york City. In 1912 she married Harold Stewart McPherson. They had a son, Rolf, but Aimee was miserable as a conventional wife. She was often ill and felt that God was punishing her for putting her evangelism aside.

In 1915 she left her husband and returned with her children to her hometown of Ingersoll. Although the couple briefly reconciled, they separated permanently in 1918 and were divorced in 1921. At home she began once again to conduct revivals. Soon she took her program on the road, where it grew in prominence and size. Her mother came along as a manager.

After several years of touring, McPherson settled in Los Angeles, where she built her Angelus Temple. Her upbeat, positive preaching attracted thousands of followers, and soon she had built an empire. The church, renamed the International Church of the Foursquare Gospel, was incorporated in 1927.

> *A different kind of "healer," the controversial evangelist ran a number of philanthropic enterprises before her empire collapsed.*

The organization's charitable works were formidable. She involved her myriad followers as volunteers in organizations including a free employment bureau, summer camps, round-the-clock prayer groups, a hotline for spiritually troubled congregants, and the Commissary, which provided food and clothing to the poorest members.

In 1926 McPherson caused a scandal when she reappeared a month after disappearing during a swim in the Pacific. She showed up in Mexico, claiming to have been kidnapped. Many contemporaries and at least one biographer expressed their skepticism—the biographer speculated that her disappearance was a kind of vacation from her sprawling empire. She and her mother were indicted on charges of obstructing justice when the police decided that her story was a lie, but the charges were eventually dropped because of the lack of evidence.

After 1928, when McPherson became estranged from her mother, a number of misfortunes befell her. Her third marriage lasted only four years, and she was plagued by a string of lawsuits. In 1936 she also became estranged from her daughter, Roberta. She died in an Oakland, California, hotel room under mysterious circumstances in 1944, ruled an accidental overdose of sleeping pills.

TO FIND OUT MORE . . .

- McPherson, Aimee. *This Is That: Personal Experiences, Sermons, and Writings.* New York: Garland, 1985.

- Mavity, Nancy Barr. *Sister Aimee.* Garden City, NY: Doubleday, Doran, 1931.

- Sicherman, Barbara, and Carol Hurd Green, eds. *Notable American Women: The Modern Period. A Biographical Dictionary.* Cambridge, MA: The Belknap Press of Harvard University Press, 1980.

- Vernoff, Edward, and Rima Shore. *The International Dictionary of 20th Century Biography.* New York: NAL Books, 1987.

Ynes Mexia, 1870–1938

Ynes Mexia was a sort of bounty hunter of botany, venturing into remote, unexplored regions of South and Central America in search of specimens of all kinds: rare high-altitude palm trees, plants used to poison fishhooks, and (once) a blueberry-like poisonous plant that she made the painful mistake of eating. Although she only began collecting at the late age of fifty-five, Mexia gathered hundreds of thousands of specimens in the years before her death at age sixty-eight.

Mexia had a complicated childhood that left her with deep scars and a rather prickly personality. She grew up mostly on her father's land in Limestone County, Texas, with brief periods spent in Ontario, Maryland, and Philadelphia. She considered becoming a nun, but her father's will stipulated that if she entered the convent she would lose her share of his estate. Instead, at twenty-eight years old, she married a twenty-three-year-old Mexico City merchant, Herman Lane. When her father, Enrique Mexia, died a year later, his will was the subject of a bitter and protracted court battle that drew in her brother and Enrique's mistress and daughter, Amada. In the end Ynes won, but shared the money with Amada and her stepsister.

In 1904 Lane died. Four years later Mexia made a brief but nasty marriage to a twenty-two year old man, which resulted in a nervous breakdown. She moved to San Francisco, at first for therapy and then permanently, and dissolved the marriage. Around 1920 she began to fight depression by taking hiking trips with the Sierra Club, and studied botany at the University of California at Berkeley. Her mentor in collecting was **Alice Eastwood**, who taught her how to preserve her specimens. She took her first collecting trip to Mexico in 1925.

In 1926 she left for a much more extensive trip to Mexico, where she spent seven months battling tiny, burr-like ticks, panthers, biting flies, and slushy mud to collect thirty-three thousand specimens from tropical jungles, sandy streambeds, and rocky mountains all over Mexico. After a year in California, she headed out again, this time to Brazil with agrostologist **Mary Agnes**

Meara Chase. They got on each other's nerves. Chase considered herself a meticulous scientist; Mexia thought of herself as an intrepid explorer. They soon went their separate ways.

In 1929 Mexia set out on a daringly ambitious trip through Brazil up the Amazon. She went via steamship for the first twenty-five thousand miles, landing in Iquitos, Peru, then hired three Peruvian men, José, Valentíno, and Neptali, to take her another five thousand miles into Peru. They traveled via dugout canoe to the Pongo, where they were halted in their tracks by torrential rains. The four camped out for three months, fashioning thatched huts and becoming friendly with the local Aguaruna Indians, who traded food with them. When the rains abated somewhat, they helped Mexia build a balsa raft for her return trip.

Mexia found the raft exciting, but it was a dangerous way to travel in the rain-swollen river. Still she returned safely with her sixty-five thousand specimens. Another epic trip in 1933 to Ecuador found Mexia traveling up nearly vertical slopes in pursuit of ivory nut palm trees on Volcán de Chiles, slogging through belly-deep mud on oxback, and accidentally eating fiery blue-

In 1929, she set out on an ambitious trip up the Amazon to gather specimens.

berry-like berries when food ran short. The year-long trip resulted in five thousand new specimens.

Back in the United States in 1937, Mexia ignored chest pain as best she could. Another trip to Mexico was planned in October, but was cut short by illness in May of 1938. She died in a California hospital less than two months later, but not before she had brought back her final thirteen thousand plant trophies.

TO FIND OUT MORE ...

- Bonta, Margaret Meyers. *Women in the Field: America's Pioneering Naturalists*. College Station, TX: Texas A&M University Press, 1991.

- Goodspeed, T. Harper. *Plant Hunters in the Andes*. New York: Farrar and Rinehart, 1941.

- Mexia's papers are in the University and Jepson Herbaria at the University of California at Berkeley, and at the Botany Gray Herbarium at Harvard University.

Ann Haven Morgan, 1882–1966

Variously known as "Mayfly Morgan" and "the Water Bug Lady" by affectionate and amused acquaintants, Ann Haven Morgan had two careers in science. In the first, she headed the zoology department at Mount Holyoke College in Western Massachusetts. In the second, really an extension of her teaching career, she became an ardent conservationist who, like **Rachel Carson**, won over converts by making them love nature as much as she did.

Christened Anna Haven Morgan (she later changed her name to Ann) in Waterford, Connecticut, she had an early love for nature that she indulged in the nearby fields and wooded areas. She matriculated at Wellesley College in 1902 but soon transferred to Cornell University. On her graduation with a bachelor's degree in 1906, she was hired as an assistant in zoology at Mount Holyoke College in South Hadley, Massachusetts.

Mount Holyoke was Morgan's lifelong professional home. She became an instructor soon after her hiring and moved up the ranks in short order after returning to Cornell for her doctorate on mayflies, becoming an associate professor in 1914, the chairman of the zoology department in 1916, and a full professor in 1918, at the age of thirty-six. Morgan was a memorable teacher who dressed in an old-fashioned shirtwaist, tie, and long skirt whether in the classroom or in the field. At some point in her work at Mount Holyoke, she took up residence near campus with a younger professor of zoology, A. Elizabeth Adams.

Morgan made conservation an explicit goal of her work in zoology. Mayflies were a major subject of her research for that very reason. "Her favorite preoccupation has been and . . . will always be mayflies," wrote a reporter for *Time* magazine, "because mayflies are fine for small boys to fish with." If people became interested in wildlife, the reasoning went, then they would be less likely to carelessly destroy it. Morgan's particular gift lay in making her subjects, creatures that lived in mud and brackish ponds, interesting to laypeople. Her crowning accomplishment was the vivid, enthusiastic *A Field Book of Ponds and Streams*, published in 1930.

In 1933 she was one of three women featured in that year's edition of *American Men of Science*. Gradually she became more active in conservation work, leading a workshop for teachers at Goddard Park in Rhode Island in the summer of 1945. She began to collect honors and awards, including fellowships at Harvard, Yale and Cornell, and election as a fellow of the American Association for the Advancement of Science.

> *Morgan made conservation an explicit goal of her work in zoology.*

Morgan retired from the chairmanship of the zoology department at Mount Holyoke in 1947 at the age of sixty-five and traveled with Elizabeth Adams to the western United States and Canada, where they investigated approaches to conservation in those areas. Morgan was impressed with what she saw, and determined to bring more awareness to the East Coast.

To that end she focused on getting courses on ecology included in the regular school curriculum, with the idea that love of nature needed to be instilled in all Americans if we are to have any hope of preserving it. "Now that the wilderness is almost gone," she wrote in her last book, *Kinships of Animals and Man: A Textbook of Animal Biology* (1955), "we are beginning to be lonesome for it. We shall keep a refuge in our minds if we conserve the remnants."

Ann Morgan died in 1966, just as ecological awareness began to stir in America.

TO FIND OUT MORE ...

- Alexander, Charles P. "Ann Haven Morgan, 1882–1966." *Eatonia* 8 (1967): 1-3.

- Bonta, Margaret Meyers. *Women in the Field: America's Pioneering Naturalists.* College Station, TX: Texas A&M University Press, 1991.

- Morgan's papers are at the Williston Memorial Library/Archives, Mount Holyoke College, and in the Woman's Rights Collection at the Schlesinger Library at Radcliffe College.

Margaret Morse Nice, 1883–1974

Ornithologist Margaret Morse Nice turned her lifelong love of birds into serious scholarly study. Although she never earned a doctorate and worked from her home while caring for her five children, her work was of such high caliber that her fellow ornithologists welcomed her as one of their own, electing her the first woman president of the Wilson Ornithological Society in 1938 and 1939. Ethologist Konrad Lorentz noted that she had been the first to conduct a long-term study of an individual wild creature in its natural habitat.

Margaret Morse grew up on the campus of Amherst College in western Massachusetts, where scholarly influences molded her birdwatching habit into a discipline at a young age. At twelve she included articles on them in the weekly paper she wrote, "Fruit Acre News." She attended private schools and became the third woman in her mother's line to attend Mount Holyoke College.

She graduated in 1906 after completing her coursework in the natural sciences, and continued her studies as a fellow in biology at Clark University in Worcester, Massachu-

setts. There, in accordance with her parents' wishes, she met and married a nice young man, Leonard Blaine Nice, in 1909. In 1911, she followed him to Harvard Medical School. The couple moved again in 1913 to Norman, Oklahoma, where he directed the physiology department at the University of Oklahoma. Over the course of fourteen years, they had five daughters.

Meanwhile, Margaret Nice was conducting research on her own. "The Food of the Bob-White," her first article, based on over two years of careful fieldwork, was published in the *Journal of Economic Entomology* in 1910. She was given a master's degree from Clark in 1915, after her published study of the food habits of bobwhites attracted widespread attention.

While her children were young, she directed her scientific energies toward them, studying child psychology and writing articles about child development. Oklahoma bird life increasingly drew her attention, however, and she spent more and more time observing birds and recording their behavior. Between 1920 and 1960, Nice published over 240 works, including her 1924 *The Birds of Oklahoma,* the first definitive study of the region. Her children grew to be a great help in her research, climbing trees to check nests for her and delighting in the birds she often took into their home. A visitor to the house remembered being distracted by wild birds that felt free to perch on plates or on guests at dinner.

In 1927 the family of seven moved to Columbus, Ohio, when Blaine Nice got a job at Ohio State University. Columbus was the site of Margaret Nice's pioneering work on the song sparrow. She carefully labeled the birds with bands of different colors so that she could positively identify an individual from a distance. That way she was able to name and observe individuals, recording their strikingly different personalities. This pioneering study, set apart by her meticulous observations of individuals, established her as a leader in behavioral studies. "Almost single-handedly," said Ernst Mayr, she "initiated a new era in American ornithology."

Most of her writing after 1936 was done on her observations in Oklahoma and Ohio, since the family moved that year to Chicago for Blaine Nice's job at the Chicago Medical School. The city was not conducive to observations of birds in a natural habitat. Nice expanded her interests to conservation when her love of birds made her speak out in print and on radio against pesticides and abuses of wildlife preserves.

Illness slowed her down in later years, but she continued to pursue her own research and to publish late in life. As always, she was supported by her husband, who enjoyed her success and popularity in ornithology as much as she did. She was an associate editor of the journal *Bird-Banding* until her death at age ninety, a few months after her husband died.

> *An accomplished amateur ornithologist, Nice was the first to conduct a long-term study of an individual wild creature in its natural habitat.*

TO FIND OUT MORE . . .

- Bonta, Margaret Meyers. *Women in the Field: America's Pioneering Naturalists.* College Station, TX: Texas A&M University Press, 1991.

- Sicherman, Barbara, and Carol Hurd Green, eds. *Notable American Women: The Modern Period. A Biographical Dictionary.* Cambridge, MA: The Belknap Press of Harvard University Press, 1980.

Elsie Clews Parsons, 1875–1941

A nthropologist, sociologist, and folklorist Elsie Parsons was a woman scientist who used her science to underline her feminism and contradict some widely held beliefs about women. She also successfully combined motherhood with an active scientific career and her position as the wife of a Republican congressman. Her straightforward explorations of taboo subjects, like the sexual practices of different religions and the barriers of age, gender, and class in early twentieth-century America, were sometimes published under a pseudonym to protect her husband's career from the backlash against her books.

Elsie Clews was born in New York City, where her father had founded a banking firm. Her mother, Lucy Madison Clews, was a Southerner who counted President Madison among her ancestors. The Clewses were socially prominent, and Elsie's mother had hoped that her only daughter would undertake a life of leisure, but instead she enrolled at Barnard after graduating from private school.

In 1896 she went on to pursue a Ph.D. in sociology at Columbia University, earning her degree in 1899. Columbia published her dissertation later that year. She married a New York lawyer and alderman, Herbert Parsons, in Newport, Rhode Island in 1900. They had six children together over the next ten years, four of whom lived to adulthood.

Meanwhile, Elsie Parsons did not slow her academic career. She was a lecturer at Barnard and taught a course at Columbia University. Her first popular book, *The Family*, was published in 1906. In it, she argued that equal professional opportunities for women made them better wives and mothers. In 1906, quite the reverse was generally believed to be the case, and feminists thankfully seized on her explanations of the sociological roots of the subjugation of women.

The book also promoted the idea of

trial marriage, which drew quite a bit of flak from conservative readers. The political fallout from the controversy was used to great effect by opponents of Herbert Parsons, so the next time Elsie Parsons had something controversial to write (*Religious Chastity*, 1913), she published under the name John Main. Other less scandalous but equally witty and feminist books followed, under her own name, yearly through 1916: *The Old-Fashioned Woman* (1913), *Fear and Conventionality* (1914), *Social Freedom* (1915), and *Social Rule* (1916). Her mother was appalled by Elsie's public position.

> **Her writings, which promoted the idea of trial marriage, sparked intense controversy.**

Her attention shifted to Native American culture after a trip with her husband to the Southwest in 1915. She left her oldest daughter, Lissa, in charge of the younger children and began a long period of field trips that took her away from home to study the Zuñi, Taos, Laguna, Hopi, and Tewa people in Arizona and New Mexico. In the course of her anthropological work, she became interested in folklore. She traveled to Ecuador, the Caribbean, the Massachusetts coast, and the Antilles, recording folktales from different cultures.

All this time she published prolifically, writing about ten more books and over a hundred articles for scholarly publications. After Herbert Parsons died in 1925, she extended her trips and devoted even more time to her work. She was active until her death in 1940, conducting research, publishing regularly, and serving terms as president of organizations including the American Folklore Society and the American Anthropological Association. She died in New York City in 1941, at age sixty-five.

TO FIND OUT MORE ...

- Hare, Peter. *A Woman's Quest for Science: A Portrait of Anthropologist Elsie Clews Parsons.* Buffalo, NY: Prometheus Books, 1985.

- Ogilvie, Marilyn Bailey. *Women in Science.* Cambridge, MA: The MIT Press, 1986.

- Sicherman, Barbara, and Carol Hurd Green, eds. *Notable American Women: The Modern Period. A Biographical Dictionary.* Cambridge, MA: The Belknap Press of Harvard University Press, 1980.

- Parsons' papers are at the Schlesinger Library at Radcliffe College, and in the library of the American Philosophical Society.

Edith Patch, 1876–1954

When entomologist Edith Patch was hired to teach entomology at the University of Maine, one man challenged her employer for hiring a woman. "Why on earth did you do that?" he complained. "A *woman* can't catch grasshoppers." Her employer, who knew better, retorted, "It will take a lively grasshopper to escape Miss Patch." Actually it was aphids that did not escape Edith Patch. She became an international authority on aphids of all sorts.

Patch was the boisterous youngest child of six born in Worcester, Massachusetts. After her family moved to prairie property near Minneapolis, Minnesota, when she was eight, she brought her interest in nature to school. An essay written on monarch butterflies won her twenty-five dollars—a princely sum which she used to buy the scholarly tome *Manual for the Study of Insects*, written by John Henry Comstock and illustrated by his wife, **Anna Botsford Comstock**.

Like **Rachel Carson**, Patch was a born writer but a scientist by profession. As an undergraduate at the University of Minnesota she studied English and won prizes for her sonnets, but on her graduation in 1901, she began to search for jobs in entomology. She ran into plenty of resistance from people who told her sniffingly that entomology was *not* a field for a woman, but after two years of supporting herself on an English teacher's salary, she found one receptive letter from Charles D. Woods at the University of Maine. He was looking for someone to head the entomology department he wanted to organize, and he was willing to take her on—at no pay—for a year to see whether she would measure up. She jumped at the chance.

Woods quickly saw that his protegee was more than up to the job, and awarded her a salary and a teaching position. Ignoring the protests of sexist colleagues, he made her the head of the department in 1904. She spent the rest of her professional life in that position. Early on she took advantage of her situation to finish her scientific education, earning a master's degree from Maine in 1910. She was thrilled to be able to finish her doctorate at Columbia under J.H. Comstock, who regarded her with warmth and pride as an outstanding student. Later he used part of her thesis for his *Introduction to Entomology*. Anna Comstock was impressed with the books she wrote for children on entomology, which were at once meticulously correct and entertaining.

Meanwhile, she had begun research on the habits of aphids. Most aphids live and feed on only one species of plant, and they can be a plague to farmers of their host plant. One of Patch's most important discoveries was that the melon aphid spent its winters as an egg in the "live-for-ever weed". Eliminating the weed could significantly limit the damage the aphids could inflict on the crops.

> *Edith Patch's extensive knowledge of aphids put her in great demand. Researchers from all over the world sent her specimens.*

Her knowledge put her in great demand among researchers, who sent her aphid specimens from all over the world. Her expertise finally overcame lingering sexism when the Entomological Society of America made her its president in 1930. One male colleague wrote her a letter of congratulations in which he deplored the lateness of the appointment. "The fact that you are not a man," he said, "was the only excuse."

She continued to write in lucid prose for both children and adults. Her *Food Plant Catalogue of the Aphids* was an enormous and exhaustive work, a major contribution to entomology, but she may have had a more lasting impact with her wonderful and popular children's stories of nature. She retired in the late thirties. Royalties from her books and her pension from the University of Maine supported her in comfort, but after her sister died in the late forties, Patch had a rather sad life. Lonely and without companionship, she would give strangers on buses candy bars in hopes of a little conversation, and she often showed up at the houses of acquaintances unexpectedly around dinnertime in search of friendship. She did befriend a doctor after a bout of pneumonia, and she left her belongings to him and his wife after her death in 1954.

TO FIND OUT MORE . . .

- Bonta, Margaret Meyers. *Women in the Field: America's Pioneering Naturalists.* College Station, TX: Texas A&M University Press, 1991.

- Patch's papers are at the Raymond H. Folger Library at the University of Maine.

Cecilia Payne-Gaposchkin, 1900–1979

. . . .

Born with the century, research astronomer Cecilia Payne-Gaposchkin would become one of the first notable women to deal with a thorny problem: juggling the demands of career and those of family.

Cecilia Payne was born to a family of intellectuals living outside London. Both Cecilia and her sister Leonora spent their undergraduate years studying to enter professions. Leonora became an architect and Cecilia, unable to find a position in astronomy in England, set off for the Harvard Observatory in Cambridge, Massachusetts.

Like any woman graduate student at Harvard at the time, she was required to enroll at Radcliffe. She wrote a brilliant dissertation on the composition and temperature of stellar atmospheres, earning her doctorate from Radcliffe in 1925. Reluctantly—for again there were no positions to be found for women in England—she stayed on at Harvard, first as a postdoctoral fellow and later as a member of the permanent staff.

She was able to pursue her research on the atmospheric makeup of stars as a post-doctoral fellow, but when she joined the staff, her research had to follow the Observatory's priorities. After a few years of chafing in her narrowly defined role as a staff member, Payne began serious work on variable stars. In 1933 she co-authored two papers on novae and nebulae. Encouraged by her colleagues, she prepared for a research trip to Europe.

Payne was appalled to find her Eastern European counterparts working in poverty. When she met the Russian emigre Sergei Gaposchkin in Berlin, she immediately sympathized with his drive to leave his current position—for political reasons, his position at Berlin University was imperiled—and began trying to find him a position at Harvard. Her efforts won him a position as a research assistant there. Soon after he arrived, they slipped away to New York to be married, an act that surprised her friends at the Observatory; they saw it as eloping. Still, when the couple returned, they were enthusiastically welcomed back into the Observatory community.

Payne-Gaposchkin made her intention to continue an active career clear from the start; she chose to hyphenate her name so that her writings might be more easily found by those who sought them. As a mother of three she was equally uncompromising about her family life. Child care, particularly, was a constant obstacle. After some difficult experiences with nannies, the Gaposchkins began to take their children to the Observatory, where, often to the consternation of their colleagues, the children spent much of their early years. Meanwhile, Payne-Gaposchkin pressed on with her research on variable stars.

> *After some difficult experiences with nannies, the Gaposchkins began to take their children to the Harvard Observatory.*

The Gaposchkins, congenial co-workers, collaborated on a series of publications. Gaposchkin's career was boosted by his wife's; she was widely regarded as the superior scientist. He would eventually, however, prove to be a detriment to her career. Despite her obvious accomplishments, one Harvard colleague declined to recommend her for the presidency of Bryn Mawr College, citing her husband's personality as problematic. (The colleague may also have been angling to keep her at Harvard). Still, she thrived at Harvard, becoming the first woman to recieve tenure there (in 1956) and the first woman to chair its department of astronomy. She remained on the Harvard Observatory staff until her death in 1979.

Payne-Gaposchkin was passionate about both her work and her family—otherwise she might not have managed both—but her work was her first true love, and one she only left when confined by pregnancy. In her autobiography, she wrote a poem that appears at the end of the book. It is titled "Research."

> *O Universe, O Lover*
> *I gave myself to thee*
> *Not for gold*
> *Not for glory*
> *But for love.*

TO FIND OUT MORE . . .

- Abir-Am, Pnina, and Dorinda Outram, eds. *Uneasy Careers and Intimate Lives: Women in Science, 1789–1979*. New Jersey: Rutgers, The State University, 1987.

- Payne-Gaposchkin, Cecilia. *An Autobiography and Other Recollections*. Cambridge, 1984.

Mary Engle Pennington, 1872–1952

M ary Engle Pennington became a chemist around the turn of the century. It was a difficult time to be a woman in a scientific field, and Pennington ran into a fair amount of opposition. The sheer excellence of her work, however, made it difficult for people to ignore her. To get a job with the Department of Agriculture, she slipped by as M.E. Pennington until she had become indispensable to her department. Her work there in food preservation methods made refrigeration possible.

Mary was born in Nashville, Tennessee, but when she was very young her Quaker parents moved the family to Philadelphia. Her parents were not strict Quakers; they did not oppose her when she decided to apply for admission to the University of Pennsylvania's Towne Scientific School. She got in, but when she had completed the requirements for a B.S., the university refused to grant her one and instead gave her a certificate of proficiency in 1892.

Undaunted, Pennington continued her graduate work at the University of Pennsylvania, earning her Ph.D. in chemistry in 1895. She found on graduation that jobs in chemistry were hard to come by for women. After three years as a graduate fellow in chemistry and botany at Pennsylvania and Yale, she decided to open her own business. Her Philadelphia Clinical Laboratory served area physicians, performing bacteriological analyses on the samples they sent her.

She quickly made a name for herself in the Philadelphia medical community, and she was asked to head the city health department's bacteriological lab and lecture at the Woman's Medical College of Pennsylvania. Harvey Wiley, an old family friend and the head of the Department of Agriculture's chemistry bureau, kept track of her success, and in 1905 he approached her about the possibility of her working on his food preservation project. He advised her to sign her exams "M.E. Pennington" to keep the Department from questioning the hiring of a woman. In 1907 she got the job and was made chief of the Food Research Laboratory only a year later.

In prerefrigeration days, Pennington's work on methods of food preservation were extremely important. Spoiled food often poisoned unlucky consumers. When refrigeration was first introduced, it sucked all the moisture out of the food, rendering it inedible. Early attempts to humidify the air went too far and made the food inedibly moldy. It was Pennington who developed a method of controlling the humidity and making refrigeration workable. For her devotion to her research, she earned a Notable Service Medal.

> *Pennington's work on methods of food preparation had important public health ramifications in the days before refrigeration.*

Pennington left the Department of Agriculture in 1919 and struck out on her own once more, setting up a lucrative consulting business in New York. She spent much of her time visiting packing houses and warehouses across the United States. She became interested in frozen foods, and delighted in serving them (thawed, of course) to friends. She continued to work at her consulting business until her death at age eighty. When she died, she was the vice president of the American Institute of Refrigeration.

TO FIND OUT MORE . . .

- Sicherman, Barbara, and Carol Hurd Green, eds. *Notable American Women: The Modern Period. A Biographical Dictionary.* Cambridge, MA: The Belknap Press of Harvard University Press, 1980.

- Vare, Ethlie Ann, and Greg Ptacek. *Mothers of Invention: From the Bra to the Bomb, Forgotten Women and Their Unforgettable Ideas.* New York: William Morrow, 1988.

- Yost, Edna. *American Women of Science.* New York: J.B. Lippincott Company, 1955.

Susan La Flesche Picotte, 1865–1915

. . . .

Susan La Flesche Picotte, the youngest of five children of an Omaha chief, was a physician and activist who returned home to Nebraska after her East Coast education to work as a doctor and carry on her father's temperance work on the Omaha reservation where she was born. She lobbied for laws to control alcohol on reservations, and founded a hospital that was named for her after her death.

The La Flesche family was a remarkably active one. Susan's father, Joseph La Flesche (Iron Eye), worked to stamp out the alcoholism that he saw undermining his reservation's people, and he passed that cause on to all five of his children. Susan was educated until age fourteen on the reservation, in the government and missionary schools set up for Native American children.

At fourteen she left home for New Jersey, where, like her older sister Suzette, she attended the Elizabeth Institute for Young Ladies. She continued her education at the Hampton Institute in Virginia, where she excelled, graduating second in her class and winning a medal for her academic accomplishments. A philanthropic organization helped to provide tuition for medical school at the Woman's Medical College of Pennsylvania; this time she graduated first in her class.

La Flesche interned for a year at the Woman's Hospital in Philadelphia before returning to the Omaha reservation, from which she had been away for over a decade. She found a position as the doctor for the government school there, but her services were soon in demand from the whole tribe. La Flesche untiringly attended to the needs of her reservation, traveling via horseback to cover the huge range of her patient population.

In 1894 she married Henry Picotte (half French, half Sioux) and moved with him to Bancroft, Nebraska. He died after a debilitating illness in 1905, and she raised their two boys on her own, making sure both attended college. Throughout their childhood she continued to practice medicine for both her white and her Native American neighbors.

In 1906, the town of Walthill was founded on Susan Picotte's reservation. She went to Washington, D.C., with other Native American leaders to push for legislation banning the sale of alcohol in all towns on the Winnebago and Omaha reservations. The delegation was successful.

> *La Flesche untiringly attended to the needs of her reservation, traveling via horseback to cover the huge range of her patient population.*

According to the biographer of the La Flesche family, Susan Picotte became the unofficial leader of the Omaha tribe. She had treated every member of the tribe until her death in 1915, and in 1913 she established a hospital in Walthill, named for her after her death. Her final years were made painful by an infection of her facial bones to which she finally succumbed in 1915 at the age of fifty.

TO FIND OUT MORE . . .

- Brown, Marion Marsh. *Homeward the Arrow's Flight.* Abingdon, 1980.

- Green, Norma Kidd. *Iron Eye's Family: The Children of Joseph La Flesche.* 1969.

- Sicherman, Barbara, and Carol Hurd Green, eds. *Notable American Women: The Modern Period. A Biographical Dictionary.* Cambridge, MA: The Belknap Press of Harvard University Press, 1980.

Hortense Powdermaker, 1896–1970

ortense Powdermaker grew up in a Jewish family in Pennsylvania. Highly sensitive to social distinctions, she used her finely tuned antennae to investigate race relations in the United States as an anthropologist in the 1930s and 1940s.

Powdermaker was born in Philadelphia, the daughter of second-generation German-Jewish parents. The family moved to Reading, Pennsylvania, when she was still very young, and settled in Baltimore, Maryland, when she was about twelve. As a teenager she turned her social sensibilities on her parents, rejecting their capitalist values. (Both parents' families made their money in business.) At Goucher College, her socialist leanings were further cemented when, as a Jew, she was not asked to join a sorority. On her graduatiion in 1919 she worked in New York City for the Amalgamated Clothing Workers, becoming a union leader.

While taking classes at the London School of Economics, she found her voca-tion in an anthropology class. Her professor, Bronislaw Malinowski, took her on as a graduate student and became her mentor. She graduated with a Ph.D. from the University of London in 1928 and began conducting field studies a year later. She spent ten months in the Pacific Islands, publishing her study on New Ireland, *Life in Lesu,* in 1933.

From 1930 to 1937, Powdermaker worked with the Institute of Human Relations at Yale University. One of her projects during this period was a study of Indianola, Mississippi, conducted between 1932 and 1934. During her time there, she helped psychologist John Dollard get started on his study of the town. Although Dollard pre-empted Powdermaker by publishing his study on Indianola first, Powdermaker's study was more thorough. Its exploration of the social structures of the white and black communities of the town are especially illuminating.

In 1938 Queens College hired her as an

instructor in anthropology. Powdermaker founded a joint anthropology and sociology program at Queens and taught there for the next three decades, becoming a full professor in 1954. Her lectures were popular. She had a knack for reaching students, which she put to good use in her 1944 book for high schoolers, *Probing Our Prejudices*.

Powdermaker continued to explore issues of race with articles like "The Anthropological Approach to the Problem of Modifying Race Attitudes" (*Journal of Negro Education*, Summer 1944). In 1946 and 1947, however, she turned her attention to Hollywood, where she spent two years researching her famous *Hollywood, The Dream Factory* (1950). The pioneering study criticized the way the values of the insular Hollywood community shaped the movies produced there. Around 1960 Powdermaker took her experience in mass media to northern Rhodesia (now Zambia), where she explored the relationship between social change and the media. Her findings were published in *Copper Town* (1962).

Two years before her retirement from Queens College, Powdermaker published her last work, *Stranger and Friend: The Way of an Anthropologist*, memoir of her experiences in field research. She was doing post-retirement work on women and culture when she died at the age of seventy-three.

> **Her pioneering study criticized the way the values of the insular Hollywood community shaped popular entertainment.**

TO FIND OUT MORE ...

- Powdermaker, Hortense. *Stranger and Friend: The Way of an Anthropologist*. 1966.

  - Sicherman, Barbara, and Carol Hurd Green, eds. *Notable American Women: The Modern Period. A Biographical Dictionary*. Cambridge, MA: The Belknap Press of Harvard University Press, 1980.

- Obituary. The *New York Times*, July 23, 1968.

Ida Cohen Rosenthal, 1886–1973

. . . .

Ida Rosenthal wasn't a scientist in the strict sense, but like **Bette Nesmith Graham**, she was an inventor whose creation has played a small role in many lives. As a designer in a New York dress shop in the 1920s, she created the brassiere to flatter her customers' figures for the straight, swingy flapper styles that were then popular. A canny businesswoman, she incorporated the immensely profitable Maidenform Company with her husband in 1923.

Ida was born Ida Kaganovitch near Minsk, Russia. Her family fled the country in 1904, when the Czarist regime threatened their way of life. The Kaganovitches emigrated to America, where they changed their name to the less foreign-sounding Cohen. The twenty-year old Ida worked in Hoboken, New Jersey, as a seamstress in her own tiny shop. In 1906 she married William Rosenthal.

Rosenthal joined her in the management of the shop, which profited from the growing demand for ready-to-wear clothes. The shop moved to Manhattan and became a modest success, employing twenty workers. Ida invested in a chic midtown dress shop in the early twenties, where she first developed the modern bra.

An earlier version had been patented by Caresse Crosby in 1914, the "backless brassiere." This contraption squashed the breasts flat against a woman's ribcage, and was a great improvement over the confining—often debilitating—corsets that could, in extreme cases, asphyxiate the wearer. Many of Rosenthal's customers, however, were far too top-heavy for Cohen's creation to do them much good. To make her flippy dresses sit more flatteringly on their curvy figures, she designed a new garment that gave support without crushing her customers' chests, and gave it away with her dresses to improve sales.

Rosenthal's gimmick was enormously successful as a sales tool, but she realized

THE REMARKABLE LIVES OF

that she was sitting on a gold mine when they began to return to buy the gimmick without the dresses. Ida and William Rosenthal moved quickly to start up the Maidenform Company in 1923. They used their savings—$4,500—to found it, an investment that proved a wise one. By 1938 the company was grossing one thousand times that amount annually; in the late 1960s the annual gross was more like ten thousand times the original investment.

Rosenthal's husband, an amateur sculptor, came up with the idea that led to the cup size system that now is standard in all brassieres. He was Maidenform's head of production; Ida was the treasurer and handled sales and advertising for many years. When William died in 1958, she became the company's president. She remained an active representative for Maidenform almost until her death in her eighty-seventh year.

> *Her invention launched the immensely successful Maidenform Company in 1923.*

TO FIND OUT MORE . . .

- Vare, Ethlie Ann, and Greg Ptacek. *Mothers of Invention: Forgotten Women and Their Unforgettable Ideas.* New York: William Morrow & Co., 1988.

Jane Anne Russell, 1911–1967

I ronically, biochemist Jane Anne Russell's career illustrated both the heights women could reach and the barriers they faced in medicine in the 1940s and 1950s. Despite her well-recognized pioneering research in carbohydrate metabolism in the late 1930s, Russell was not recognized with a full professorship until 1965, only two years before her death of breast cancer.

Russell was the baby in a family of five children born to Mary Ann Phillips Russell and Josiah Howard Russell. The family lived near Los Angeles, California, where Josiah eked out a living for his large family as a rancher and deputy sheriff. Jane Russell went to Polytechnic High School for the last two years of high school, graduating second in her class. She then went on to college at the University of California at Berkeley, where she graduated first in her class and was showered with awards.

After her graduation in 1932, Russell enrolled at Berkeley as a graduate student in biochemistry. During her first year she supported herself with a lab job, but soon won fellowships to pay for her training. She wrote her doctoral thesis on the relationship between pituitary hormones and carbohydrate metabolism, publishing six papers on the subject before she received her doctorate in 1937. She demonstrated that an unidentified pituitary factor—which she later showed to be growth hormone—kicked in when carbohydrate deprivation threatened, keeping levels of blood glucose from dropping too low. Her expertise on the subject of carbohydrate metabolism was later the basis of her brief period of work with Nobel prizewinner **Gerty Cori**.

After a year as a postdoctoral fellow at Berkeley, Jane Russell went to Yale as a National Research Council Fellow. By now she was already a recognized authority in her field, but she continued at Yale for the next twelve years as a fellow, gathering awards and citations but no academic appointments. Among her prizes was the Ciba Award in 1946, an honor usually given to full professors. Despite her lack of a formal position, Russell was tacitly recognized by those who should have been her professional peers when she served on the committee that reviewed applications for grants to the National Institute of Health (NIH) after 1949. She was also elected vice president of the Endocrine Society in 1950.

In 1940 Russell married Alfred Ellis Wilhelmi, the researcher who had discovered the growth hormone she had demonstrated to be the factor in maintaining carbohydrate levels. The couple moved to Atlanta, Georgia, in 1950, where both were hired by Emory University to work in the department of biochemistry. Wilhelmi was a full professor and the chairman of the department, and Russell—in her first academic appointment—was an assistant professor. At Emory Russell continued her groundbreaking research and prolific publishing—she published over seventy papers—while serving the students as an excellent teacher and role model.

Emory promoted her to associate pro-

Despite her lack of a formal position, Russell was tacitly recognized by those who should have been her professional peers when she served on the committee that reviewed applications for grants to the National Institute of Health (NIH).

fessor in 1953, but held off promoting her to a full professor for another twelve years. During that time she gathered further honors from the National Science Board and the Endocrine Society and served on selection and study committees. Like Gerty Cori, however, at least one of her honors was awarded jointly to her and her husband.

When she was finally promoted to full professorship, her breast cancer had already been diagnosed. She died two years later, at the age of fifty-six.

TO FIND OUT MORE . . .

- Sicherman, Barbara, and Carol Hurd Green, eds. *Notable American Women: The Modern Period. A Biographical Dictionary.* Cambridge, MA: The Belknap Press of Harvard University Press, 1980.

- Russell's papers are in the archives at Emory University.

Florence Rena Sabin, 1871–1953

. . . .

Florence Sabin, physician and tuberculosis expert, was a true leader in American science. In her twenty years at Johns Hopkins, she impressed students with her enthusiasm and dedication. One recalled that she tore up her notes after each lecture so that she would approach the subject fresh each year. At the Rockefeller Institute, where she spent the next thirteen years, she led a team of young researchers (many of whom themselves became eminent in their fields) who elucidated the body's response to tuberculosis infection. After her retirement at age sixty-seven, she returned to her Colorado home to spend over a decade leading the state's push for better organized and financed public-health programs.

In 1893 Sabin graduated with a B.S. from Smith College with the intention of going to medical school. It took her three years to earn enough money teaching math in Colorado and zoology at Smith, but in 1896 she enrolled in the fourth class to include women at Johns Hopkins University School of Medicine. Her mentor there was Franklin Mall, who guided her study and hired her as an assistant in anatomy after her graduation. Sabin later wrote a memoir of Mall, in which she said that she owed her career in medical science to him. Sabin published some of her findings as an undergraduate at Hopkins in *An Atlas of the Medulla and Midbrain* (1901), which became a popular textbook.

As a researcher at Hopkins, Sabin quickly gained the respect and admiration of her students, most of whom originally found a woman professor an unusual phenomenon. She also earned the respect of her colleagues for her pioneering work on the development of the lymphatic system, then believed to arise in the embryo from spaces between tissues and to grow toward blood vessels. Using dyes injected into the veins of very small pig embryos, Sabin demonstrated that the process went the other way around: the lymphatic system originated in small buds on blood vessels and spread outward from there.

Sabin was made full professor after fifteen years at Hopkins. It is probably as much a tribute to her excellent teaching skills as an indication of the University's discriminatory policies that the researcher to succeed Mall was not Sabin but an old student of hers, Lewis Weed. Still, Sabin was disappointed, and she left for the Rockefeller Institute after her election to the National Academy of Sciences in 1925. At the Rockefeller Institute, her team conducted research on the body's reaction on a cellular level to tuberculosis infection.

> *Sabin literally tore up her notes after each lecture so she would approach teaching her subject fresh each year.*

When Sabin retired in 1938 from the Institute, she took with her many honors, including honorary Sc.D. degrees from U. Penn, Oberlin, Smith, NYU, and Mount Holyoke, as well as election to several "Most Eminent Women in America" lists. She returned to her home state, Colorado, but was unable to slide quietly into retirement. Instead, she loaned her considerable talents to several organizations dedicated to improving public health measures in the state. By 1947 she was a well-known public figure,

feared by some lawmakers for her determined lobbying in favor of her cause. As the chairman of several boards, Sabin's opinion carried weight, and by the time she was awarded the prestigious Lasker Award in 1951, Colorado's public health programs were much improved.

Later that year the University of Colorado Medical School named its new Cellular Biology building after her. When she died of a heart attack at a World Series baseball game shortly before her eighty-second birthday, the University found that she had willed everything to the Medical College.

TO FIND OUT MORE ...

- Ogilvie, Marilyn Bailey. *Women in Science.* Cambridge, MA: The MIT Press, 1986.

- O'Hern, Elizabeth Moot. *Profiles of Pioneer Women Scientists.* New York: Acropolis Books, 1985.

- Sicherman, Barbara, and Carol Hurd Green, eds. *Notable American Women: The Modern Period. A Biographical Dictionary.* Cambridge, MA: The Belknap Press of Harvard University Press, 1980.

- Yost, Edna. *American Women of Science.* New York: J.B. Lippincott Company, 1955.

Margaret Sanger, 1879–1966

The nurse who led the birth control movement had strong personal reasons for believing that women should be able to control her biological destinies. Her Roman Catholic mother had borne eleven children and died at age forty-seven of tuberculosis. Her father, an idealist, was not financially successful in his stone monument business, and Margaret Sanger always felt that the burdens her mother had to bear on the tight family budget—and as a result of her own fertility—contributed to her early death. She may have had a point. Her father lived into his eighties.

After her mother died, Sanger left her father to go to nursing school in White Plains, New York, once again supported by her sisters' hard work. She was on the track to a promising career—she had won admittance at a three-year program and had two years' experience in practical nursing—when she met the architect and aspiring artist William Sanger in 1902. She apologized to her sisters; she had fallen in love with his idealism, so like her father's. They were married and had three children in seven years.

At thirty-one, Sanger felt trapped in her life as a housewife and mother of young children. In an attempt to mend their differences, the couple moved to Manhattan to work as political activists in the city. Margaret Sanger took a job as a nurse to support her work with unions, but it was her expertise as a nurse that made her a sought-after resource among her socialist friends. She moved to the forefront of the budding struggle for sexual reform, and by 1912 she was publishing public-service articles about birth control, venereal diseases, and sex education. One early article was censored under the Comstock Act of 1873, which deemed all birth control-related matters obscene.

Angered by the censorship and by the appalling situations in which she found women ignorant of medical knowledge, Sanger pushed on. She was particularly horrified by a patient who died of a self-induced abortion; she later said that this event led her to focus exclusively on the issue of biological autonomy for women. She worked for women who, she felt, were trapped by their own lack of knowledge.

Faced with a society that willfully ignored female sexuality, Sanger separated from her husband and took a trip to Europe to research methods of birth control. She returned in 1914 to New York to begin publication of her journal *The Woman Rebel*, also censored under the Comstock Act. She left the country later that same year to avoid prosecution, although the journal offered no specific advice on contraceptive methods. After a year of exile in Europe, Sanger's daughter died of pneumonia. When she returned, grieving, to New York, public sympathy for her was so strong that the government dropped the charges against her. Sanger turned again to her cause for solace.

> For Sanger, the experience of a patient who died of a self-induced abortion was the turning point.

With her younger sister, Sanger opened a clinic in Brooklyn to distribute advice on birth control. It was closed by the police in ten days. The trial made her nationally famous, and in an appeal, the New York law was clarified: A clause that permitted doctors to prescribe condoms for the prevention of disease was broadened to include women patients. Sanger used the ruling to legitimize birth control by making it an issue for professionals in medicine. In 1921, divorced from her husband, she founded the American Birth Control League which later became the Planned Parenthood Federation of America.

In 1922 she married J. Noah Slee, a wealthy man who helped fund her work and who accepted her very independent lifestyle, which included intimate relationships with other men. With his help she opened the first doctor-staffed birth control clinic, the Birth Control Clinical Research Bureau, in 1923. The doctors at the Manhattan clinic made its operation legal; Sanger's tenacity in court had paid off. In 1936 she reversed the Comstock Act in court, and in 1937 the AMA recognized contraception as a valid subject for medical schools to cover.

Sanger internationalized Planned Parenthood and saw a the birth control pill invented before her death in Tuscon in 1966.

TO FIND OUT MORE . . .

- Douglas, Emily Taft. *Margaret Sanger: Pioneer of the Future.* New York: Holt, Rhinehart and Winston, 1970.

- Sanger, Margaret. *Margaret Sanger: An Autobiography.* New York: W.W. Norton, 1938.

- Sicherman, Barbara, and Carol Hurd Green, eds. *Notable American Women: The Modern Period. A Biographical Dictionary.* Cambridge, MA: The Belknap Press of Harvard University Press, 1980.

Ida Sophia Scudder, 1870–1960

. . . .

Ida Scudder, missionary and physician, came from a long line of missionaries—her grandfather, John Scudder, had been the first American missionary in India. As a child growing up in America without her parents, Scudder resisted the idea of becoming a missionary, aspiring instead to lead a "normal" middle-class American life. But missionary work seemed to be in her blood. As a college student she visited her parents in India and watched three women die in labor in one night. The overwhelming need in India drew her to spend most of the rest of her life struggling to improve medical conditions there.

Ida Scudder was the baby of the family. She grew up with her parents and five older brothers in a mission bungalow in Vellore, South India. It was considered a dangerous place for children, with uncontrolled epidemics periodically sweeping the population and famine a constant threat. When Ida was eight the whole family moved to Nebraska,

where they spent four relatively tranquil years living on a farm. But Ida's parents went back to India in 1882, leaving her with an uncle. When the uncle left to become a missionary in Japan, the seventeen-year-old Ida was packed off to a boarding school in Massachusetts, Northfield Seminary.

At Northfield she was a popular student but wrote of her sadness and loneliness in her diary. She had not lived with her parents since she was twelve, and perhaps it was in a fit of rebellion that she rejected the idea of a missionary life. The family tradition was certainly a powerful one, however. According to one estimate, several generations of Scudders spent a combined total of 1,100 years as missionaries in India alone. Ida Scudder would herself contribute over fifty years.

A visit to her parents in Tindivanam changed her life. She was the only female available to help with three childbirths—men were not permitted to attend—and she could only watch helplessly as all three women died in labor. She returned to the United States to earn her medical degree. Three years at the Woman's Medical College of Pennsylvania and a final year at Cornell resulted in a degree in 1899, and Scudder left for India the next year, bringing with her her companion Annie Hancock, a classmate from Northfield who did evangelical work in India until her death in 1924.

In Vellore, Scudder found herself alone when her father died a few months after her arrival. The conditions were difficult: She was the only physician, her patients doubted her ability, and her office consisted only of a small room in the missionary bungalow. She set out to improve the situation. In 1902 the tiny Mary Taber Schell hospital was erected, and Scudder supplemented its services with her wide-ranging roadside clinics. She also began a nursing training program for the hospital, which in 1909 became a full-fledged school.

Despite the great improvement represented by the Schell Hospital, Scudder still felt that much more was needed in her part of India. She painstakingly raised funds for a medical school, the Union Mission Medical School, which opened in 1918. For fourteen years she acted as the only surgeon at Schell and as the administrator and only professor at her medical school. She spent another twelve years, from 1938 to 1950, fighting to save the school when a government regulation made training at institutions not affiliated with universities illegitimate. She finally succeeded when the University of Madras affiliated itself with the school.

With her victory, the eighty-year-old Scudder finally retired to a bungalow in the Indian hills, where she remained remarkably active until her death at age ninety.

> *The overwhelming need in India drew Scudder to spend most of her life struggling to improve medical conditions there.*

TO FIND OUT MORE . . .

- Sicherman, Barbara, and Carol Hurd Green, eds. *Notable American Women: The Modern Period. A Biographical Dictionary.* Cambridge, MA: The Belknap Press of Harvard University Press, 1980.

- Wilson, Dorothy. *Dr. Ida Scudder of Vellore.* New York: McGraw-Hill, 1959.

Florence Barbara Seibert, 1897–1991

I ronically, the polio that crippled Florence Seibert at age three would influence her decision to pursue chemistry instead of medicine, which was thought to be too physically strenuous for her. Her pioneering work as a chemist would help to stamp out another contemporary scourge—tuberculosis. Once the leading cause of death in the United States, tuberculosis became a rarity for many years thanks to measures like the efficient skin test that Seibert's research made possible. (Unfortunately it has begun making a comeback in recent years.)

Florence was the middle child in a close-knit Pennsylvania family of five. Both she and her older brother, Russell, were victims of a polio epidemic that was especially cruel to their town. Their parents were tremendously supportive; the family moved close to the children's school to make it easier for them to attend, and tirelessly worked with the children until they were able to walk, at first with braces and later without.

When Florence won a scholarship to Goucher College, her father was so worried about her ability to handle all the physical demands of college on her own that he went with her. Within a week he had gone home, for Florence was thriving. Seibert couldn't get enough of her classes, and had a hard time choosing between her favorite subjects. But "above all," she once said of her college years, "I learned . . . that I was not an invalid but could stand on my own two feet with a chance to make a contribution to the world."

After college came a short stint from 1918 to 1923 working with her old chemistry professor, Dr. Jessie Minor, for the war effort. During World War I, many women took the places of men who'd gone off to fight. Seibert and Minor took over the chemistry laboratory at the Hammersley Paper Mill Company. Seibert spent the time learning how to write a scientific paper and saving up her money for graduate school. When the war ended and women were no longer needed—or wanted—in what were seen as men's jobs, Florence left the lab for graduate school in biochemistry at Yale.

Seibert dove into her graduate work on pyrogenic (fever-causing) proteins. Her findings were intriguing enough that Yale allowed her stay on to analyze them. While working on this project, Seibert found that even her distilled water was sometimes pyrogenic, and therefore must have been contaminated. She designed a trap that blocked larger droplets of water in a still and made the water completely sterile.

"I learned . . . that I was not an invalid but could stand on my own two feet with a chance to make a contribution to the world."

Seibert followed up this early success with a fellowship at the University of Chicago, where she began the work on tuberculosis for which she is best remembered. While there, she received an award for her work with pyrogens. The award included $300, which she happily spent on a specially designed car that allowed her to drive with her stronger foot, and on a dog to keep her company on her rides. Newly happy and free, she turned her close attention to developing a skin test based on a yet-to-be-found antigen.

It took over fifteen years for Seibert to identify and then purify the antigen, and another several years before the test was approved for widespread use. In 1966, eight years after she had retired, it was finally made the official standard. She moved into a house designed by her brother with her younger sister, Mabel, who had been for many years her best laboratory assistant. Seibert continued to conduct research on her own, with the help of Mabel and several grants, until her death in 1991.

TO FIND OUT MORE . . .

- O'Hern, Elizabeth Moot. *Profiles of Pioneer Women Scientists.* Washington, D.C.: Acropolis Books, 1985.

- Seibert, Florence Barbara. *Pebbles on the Hill of a Scientist.* St. Petersburg: Petersburg Printing Co., 1968.

- Vare, Ethlie Ann, and Greg Ptacek. *Mothers of Invention: From the Bra to the Bomb, Forgotten Women and Their Unforgettable Ideas.* New York: William Morrow, 1988.

- Yost, Edna. *American Women of Science.* New York: J.B. Lippincott Company, 1955.

Ellen Churchill Semple, 1863-1932

Ellen Churchill Semple's work took her to remote parts of the world. She became an authority on the Mediterranean region, and was able to contribute her knowledge to the United States' preparation for the Versailles peace conference at the end of World War I.

Ellen Semple was born into a large, comfortable family of seven in Louisville, Kentucky. Her father's death, when Ellen was twelve, left her mother with five children to raise and educate. Ellen was provided with private tutors and later attended Vassar College, where she was the valedictorian of her class.

Five years after her graduation, Ellen met Freidreich Ratzel, a German anthropo-geographer, while on a European tour. She was intrigued by his ideas, and back in Louisville, began to study geography, economics, and sociology on her own. Her independent study was so impressive that Vassar granted her a master's degree for it.

Degree in hand, she traveled to Leipzig where, because of the university's policy against women enrolling, she would audit Professor Ratzel's classes.

Ratzel's theories were a jumping-off place for Semple. He taught that the characteristics of human societies are determined by their physical environments. Later in her career, Semple applied this thesis with equal enthusiasm and interest to groups in rural Kentucky and ancient Greece. In Leipzig she became a close friend of Ratzel's family and a favorite student, despite her auditor status. She absorbed his ideas and returned to Louisville to pursue her studies independently.

She made a reputation for herself with a 1901 paper she published that applied Ratzel's ideas to a cross-section of inhabitants of the Kentucky highlands. She conducted her research via horseback. She became a distinguished lecturer at institutions including Columbia, Oxford, and

Wellesley, and eventually took a permanent position at Clark University in Massachusetts as professor of anthropogeography. Her most influential work paid tribute to Ratzel in its title; it was *Influences of Geographic Environment, on the Basis of Ratzel's System of Anthropo-geography* (1911).

In 1918, a government group, dubbed "The Inquiry," was formed to anticipate and analyze possible problems at the Versailles peace conference. Semple was a consultant for the group, contributing significant research from her uniquely pertinent field. President Wilson relied on her reports on the Austro-Italian frontier and on the history of the Turkish empire.

Sadly, Semple's professional life did not end on a high note; toward the end of her career, her colleagues began to lean away from her deterministic approach. But perhaps it is fitting, since she had never been one to go along with the crowd, that Semple should end her career as independently as she conducted it. And it is beyond doubt that she had already done much for geography as an academic discipline.

> *Semple ended her career as independently as she had begun it.*

TO FIND OUT MORE . . .

- Ogilvie, Marilyn Bailey. *Women in Science.* Cambridge, Massachusetts: The MIT Press, 1986.

- Semple, Ellen Churchill. *Influences of Geographic Environment, on the Basis of Ratzel's System of Anthropo-geography.* New York: Holt, 1911.

Carolyn Wood Sherif, 1922–1982

Carolyn Wood married a Princeton psychology professor, Muzafer Sherif, when she was a psychology research assistant in his lab. Over the next several years she coauthored several works with him, although they were usually quoted as his alone. As the wife of an already established scientist, she had to work triply hard to build up her own reputation; she had first to overcome the general prejudice that confronted many women in the sciences, and then to prove that she had won her position in science.

Carolyn Wood's family weathered the Depression stoically in Indiana. Her parents told her only much later that her father, a supervisor at Purdue University and sometime science teacher, had had his salary cut three times over an eight-year period. Her mother made ladies' garments. Her father's position at Purdue made it the obvious choice for Carolyn's undergraduate education, and she was able to reduce her tuition expenses by making the "distinguished" list each term.

The Woods' support and expectations were behind each of their three children; Carolyn's older brother graduated in chemical engineering and her older sister in mathematics. Carolyn excelled in her mathematics aptitude tests but chose to pursue a liberal arts undergraduate course of study, focusing on history and literature in the classroom and on music and drama outside it. She graduated with highest honors.

America's involvement in World War II opened up graduate opportunities for women, and Wood's involvement with drama led her to graduate school in psychology when she began to speculate about the effect a play she had written had on its audience. In 1943 she enrolled at Iowa, where she was immediately fascinated by social psychology. She became interested in relationships between groups, especially when race was introduced into the mix. She was twenty-two when she earned her master's degree in 1944.

Wood landed a job with Audience Research, Inc., in Princeton, but found the research there unsatisfyingly unscientific. When her boss made a "Monday morning declaration of love" to her in his office, she quickly found herself a more suitable job by writing a Princeton psychologist whose work she admired. He suggested that she apply for a job with Muzafer Sherif, a psychologist from Turkey whose work she had also read.

Wood won the research assistantship and commuted to Columbia University in New York City for her doctoral work, since Princeton would not accept women in the 1940s, even as graduate students. At Princeton, Sherif and Wood found in each other admirable professional partners and emotional mainstays. When they were married, the skepticism of peers only made them bind more tightly together in their personal and professional lives.

Carolyn Sherif's doctorate was earned over a sixteen-year period which she spent raising three daughters, co-writing texts and articles with her husband at Yale, Princeton,

> *Sherif called the new atmosphere in scientific circles generated by the Women's Movement in the early 1970s, "like breathing fresh air after years of gasping."*

and Oklahoma University, and accumulating credits when she could. The University of Texas finally awarded her the degree in 1961. She was thirty-nine. In 1966, Sherif finally found her own tenure-track position on the faculty of Pennsylvania State University.

Sherif called the new atmosphere in scientific circles generated by the Women's Movement after 1972, "like breathing fresh air after years of gasping." The U.S. Department of Health, Education and Welfare began to investigate allegations of discrimination at Pennsylvania State University around then, resulting in the readjustment upward of Sherif's inequitable salary. The new respect accorded to Sherif and others, however, was more important to her. "I know I did not become a better social psychologist between 1969 and 1972," she wrote, "but I surely was treated as a better one."

Carolyn Wood Sherif died in 1980 at the age of sixty.

TO FIND OUT MORE . . .

- O'Connell, Agnes N., and Nancy Felipe Russo. *Models of Achievement: Reflections of Eminent Women in Psychology.*

Maud Caroline Slye, 1869–1954

. . . .

Pathologist Maud Caroline Slye found her niche in working with laboratory mice. Despite her lack of an advanced degree and her late age—thirty-nine—when she started conducting research, she was able to demonstrate that cancer was inheritable from generation to generation.

Maud Slye was the middle of three children born to Florence Alden Wheeler Slye and James Alvin Slye in Minneapolis, Minnesota, and raised in Marshaltown, Illinois. Although both parents came from old, established families, they had little money. Nevertheless, they were educated people who encouraged their daughter to study. Slye's mother had hopes that she might become a writer, like her father, but Maud was always drawn by science.

After graduating from high school in 1886, Slye spent five years as a stenographer in St. Paul, Minnesota. She was not able to save up much from her salary, and according to one account, when she entered the University of Chicago in 1895 she had only forty dollars to her name. She worked her way through school as the secretary of the university's president. She managed for three years before breaking down under the strain. After a brief period of recovery with relatives in Woods Hole, Massachusetts, on Cape Cod, she finished her bachelor's degree at Brown University in 1899.

Slye worked for six years teaching pedagogy and psychology at Rhode Island State Normal School. In 1908, an acquaintance from her time in Woods Hole offered her a very small stipend to join him at the University of Chicago as a graduate assistant in biology. She soon began her life work on the heredity of cancer with the first of many batches of lab mice. Her tiny stipend sometimes forced her to choose between feeding herself and feeding her mice, but in 1911 a position on the staff at the Sprague Memorial Institute at the University of Chicago made it possible for her to conduct research without starving.

Slye took exemplary care of her laboratory mice. She kept the lab immaculate to protect them from any diseases that might kill some of them and distort her results. She studied over 150,000 mice over three decades, keeping careful records on each one and insisting on handling them herself at every stage of the process. Slye found that inheritance did seem to be a factor in determining which mice developed cancer, while contagion did not, a theory that had then been voiced but not demonstrated by other researchers.

> *Her tiny stipend sometimes forced her to choose between feeding herself and feeding her mice.*

In 1919 she was hired to direct the Cancer Laboratory at the University of Chicago, and—lack of a graduate degree notwithstanding—in 1926 was made associate professor in pathology on the strength of her research work alone. She continued to investigate the issue of heredity in cancer, eventually coming up with the theory that, in mice that developed cancer, one genetic factor determined the type of cancer and another dictated the location of the tumor. This theory was eventually proven wrong.

Slye also came to believe that selective breeding could eventually eliminate cancer in humans when she found that she could breed cancer-free strains of mice in the laboratory. She suggested registering cancer histories in a central information bureau to achieve this end.

Slye's investigations were rewarded with honors, including an honorary doctorate from Brown University and a medal from the American Medical Association. She died in Chicago at the age of eighty-five.

TO FIND OUT MORE . . .

- McCoy, J.J. *The Cancer Lady: Maud Slye and Her Heredity Studies.* Nashville: T. Nelson, 1977.

- Sicherman, Barbara, and Carol Hurd Green, eds. *Notable American Women: The Modern Period. A Biographical Dictionary.* Cambridge, MA: The Belknap Press of Harvard University Press, 1980.

- Obituary. *The New York Times,* Sept. 18, 1954.

Cordelia Stanwood, 1865-1958

Ornithologist Cordelia Stanwood was a woman very much shaped by the her Victorian upbringing. Her first forty-one years illustrated the sad fate of some intelligent women in the late nineteenth century: She taught schoolchildren for a pittance until she was thirty-six, when she suffered a total nervous collapse. She returned, broken and poor, to her family, where she discovered ornithology. Her freelance writings quickly gained attention in the scientific world as important additions to the general body of knowledge. She also became known as an expert photographer who would spend hours waiting for an intimate shot.

Stanwood set out to become a teacher, hoping to train young minds and earn money for her family back in Maine. Indeed she was a good teacher, able to achieve an instant rapport with her pupils and gifted with her material. The pay, however, was poor—$650 a year in 1892, when she was twenty-seven. In hopes of pulling down the average $1,500 salary paid to drawing teachers, she spent a year earning her teaching qualifications, but upon her graduation there were no jobs to be found. Stanwood returned to her teaching job in Providence at a reduced salary of $600.

Until 1901 Stanwood taught school mostly around Massachusetts and Rhode Island. She always got good recommendations, but she was frustrated by her unrelieved state of poverty. In 1901 something broke down in her. Her Aunt Cordelia sent her first to a sanitarium in the Boston area, then home to her parents and younger brother.

It took a long time for her to heal. She often had anguished screaming fits, which alienated her father and brother. Her mother, however, was a great help and comfort to her. Even more important to Stanwood as time went on were her birds. In 1906 she began keeping field notes of her walks in the woods, especially of the birds' songs. They inspired truly joyful feelings in her for the first time in quite a while, and she lavished love on the birds in odes written into her notes.

Her devotion led to odd behavior at times, but resulted in painstakingly meticulous notes. When her articles began to attract attention from well-known ornithologists, she began to receive requests for her field notes. In this indirect manner, she contributed to many important catalogs of bird life. When her father died and her brother left, leaving her and her mother without support, Stanwood supplemented the tiny income from her writing with needlework and subsistence farming.

> *Stanwood supplemented the tiny income from her writing with needlework and subsistence farming.*

With the small inheritance left her by her aunt, she bought a camera and telephoto lens. She learned to build blinds and wait unmovingly for hours to get her intimate photographs, which were often bought for field guides and magazine articles. In fact, she became involved with her birds to the exclusion of everything else after her mother died in 1932. She sold stationery and Christmas cards door-to-door to supplement her income, but otherwise shut herself up in a room high in her lonely house when she was not out with her birds.

Stanwood did have friends among other ornithologists through her letters. In a letter to **Margaret Morse Nice**, Althea Sherman told of her little scheme to help Stanwood, whose articles were not earning her much money. Sherman bought several articles by Stanwood for the *Wilson Bulletin*, paying her out of her own pocket.

Pleased and surprised, Stanwood wrote Sherman that the *Bulletin* had paid her more for those articles than any publisher had paid for any of her other writings. She succeeded in eking out a living for herself until she was ninety with her many little jobs, but in 1955 she had to accept state aid in the form of a nursing home. She died there at the age of ninety-three.

TO FIND OUT MORE . . .

- Bonta, Margaret Meyers. *Women in the Field: America's Pioneering Naturalists.* College Station, TX: Texas A&M University Press, 1991.

- Richmond, Chandler. *Beyond the Spring: Cordelia Stanwood of Birdsacre.* Lamoine, ME: Latona Press, 1978.

- Papers are at the Stanwood Wildlife Sanctuary in Ellsworth, ME.

Mabel Staupers, 1890–1989

Mabel Staupers, nurse, proved herself a shrewd negotiator as the executive secretary and president of the National Association of Colored Graduate Nurses, which was founded in 1908 by **Martha Minerva Franklin**. Out of sheer necessity, the Armed Forces Nurse Corps had been integrated at the end of World War I, but during World War II the military was stubbornly refusing to grant African-American women the right to serve their country as nurses. At the same time, however, there was a shortage of nurses available to serve abroad. Staupers took advantage of the situation to wonder—publicly—why the military wasn't using the thousands of NACGN nurses at its disposal. By the end of the war, Staupers had finished the integration that had been started in World War I by **Adah Thoms**.

Mabel emigrated to the United States with her parents when she was thirteen years old. At twenty-four she moved from Harlem to Washington, D.C., to enroll at the Freedmen's Hospital School of Nursing (later absorbed into Howard University as its College of Nursing). On her graduation with honors at age twenty-seven, she married James Max Keaton. The marriage eventually failed, but Mabel's career in nursing flourished.

Like most graduate nurses, she started out as a private-duty nurse. After only a few years of this type of work, however, her talent for leadership emerged when she helped to organize the Booker T. Washington Sanitarium, Harlem's first inpatient center for African-American tuberculosis patients and one of the rare city medical centers where African-American doctors could practice medicine. In 1922, acting as the executive secretary of the Harlem tuberculosis committee of the New York Tuberculosis and Health Association, she conducted a study of the city's measures to combat the disease in Harlem. Her meticulously researched report got results.

Mabel Staupers (she married New Yorker Fritz C. Staupers in 1931) had long been involved with the NACGN when she was elected its executive secretary in 1934. Staupers and the group's president, Estelle Masse Riddle, became an efficient team in the leadership of the group, and held their respective posts together for fifteen years. When the United States entered World War II in 1941, the NACGN was ready to challenge the policy of segregation in the Armed Forces Nurse Corps.

The Army had a quota limiting the number of African-American nurses who could serve, and the Navy simply shut them out. Staupers made the quotas public, and in every appearance she made loudly stressed that the body of the NACGN was ready and willing to go to work. In conjunction with other African-American leaders, she secured meetings with military leaders to make a case for integration. By 1943 the Navy was reconsidering its position, while the Army had raised its quota from 56 to 160. In 1944 Staupers met with First Lady Eleanor Roosevelt. Roosevelt was sympathetic to the NACGN's struggle, and soon began to put gentle pressure on military officials.

When Surgeon General Norman T. Kirk announced in 1945 that the military might have to resort to a draft to fill the Nurse Corps, Staupers seized control of the situation and challenged the military's policies. She called on other nursing organizations,

> *She called on other nursing organizations, regardless of race, to write Washington and call for integration.*

regardless of race, to write Washington and call for integration. The letters and telegrams that flooded the War Department finally forced an end to both the quotas and the Navy's barrier, and less that two months after Staupers' challenge, the first African-American nurse was accepted into the Nurse Corps.

Three years later the NACGN achieved full integration of the American Nurses' Association. Estelle Riddle was made a member of the organization's board, and Staupers succeeded her as president in 1949. That year, the NACGN, which had been established with the goal of fully integrating the nursing profession in America, declared itself obsolete, its goal accomplished. Staupers oversaw the winding down of the association's activities.

For her work, Staupers was awarded the NAACP's prestigious Springarn Medal in 1951. She died at age ninety-nine.

TO FIND OUT MORE . . .

- Obituary. *The New York Times*, October 6, 1989.

- Hine, Darlene Clark. *Black Women in White: Racial Conflict and Cooperation in the Nursing Profession, 1890–1950.* Bloomington: Indiana University Press, 1989.

- Smith, Jessie Carey. *Notable Black American Women.* Detroit, MI: Gale Research Inc., 1992.

Nettie Maria Stevens, 1861–1912

When biologist Nettie Maria Stevens conducted her research (1901–1912), the links between chromosome activity and heredity had not yet been quite established. Inheritance had been examined by scientists since Gregor Mendel and his pea plants in 1866, and chromosomes had been carefully observed, but they were first explicitly linked in 1905 when Stevens documented the differences between male and female, or X and Y, chromosomes.

Nettie Maria Stevens was one of two surviving children, both girls, of Julia and Ephraim Stevens. Her father was a carpenter. She showed great academic promise as a student at the public schools near her Westford, Massachusetts, home, and completed her high school education at Westford Academy, graduating in 1880. After three more years of education at the Westfield Normal School, she graduated at the top of her class.

Stevens took the more socially accept-able path for a woman of her academic distinction in the late nineteenth century: She worked for thirteen years (1883-1896) as a librarian and schoolteacher near Westford. After spending her entire life in and around her home in Westford, however, she made a bold and sudden move: She applied to Stanford University in far-off California.

Stanford accepted her as a special student in 1896, and in 1897 she became a thirty-five-year-old freshman. Her father and sister came to live near her in California two years later. Her years at Stanford were happy and productive ones; she spent her summers studying at the Hopkins Seaside Laboratory in Pacific Grove and became gradually interested in the microscope-centered fields of histology and cytology. She earned a bachelor's degree in 1899 and a master's degree in 1900, writing a master's thesis on ciliate protozoa (microscopic organisms with small hairs that function as propellers).

In 1900 Stevens moved back East to earn her doctorate at Bryn Mawr College. It was a wonderful time to study at Bryn Mawr; Thomas Hunt Morgan, the Nobel Prize-winning geneticist, and Edmund Beecher Wilson, noted biologist, had added to the excellence of the biology department, although Wilson left before Stevens enrolled in 1900. Her brilliant work at Bryn Mawr resulted in a fellowship to study in Italy and Germany, and she earned her Ph.D. in 1903 with a dissertation that continued her investigation of ciliate protozoa.

Nettie Stevens stayed on at Bryn Mawr to work as a research fellow in biology. She began to write prolifically, publishing thirty-eight papers in her short career. In 1935 she published the paper that first linked the number of chromosomes with the sex of the organism. Her study was on mealworms. Her theory was not well received at the time; it was better accepted when later presented by Edmund Wilson, who arrived at the same conclusions some time after Stevens's untimely death of breast cancer in 1912. (To be fair, Wilson reached the same conclusions independently of, albeit somewhat after, Stevens' work.)

> *Stanford accepted her as a special student in 1896, and in 1897 she became a thirty-five-year-old freshman.*

Although her contribution is often attributed to Wilson, Stevens' scientific achievement was honored during her lifetime with the Ellen Richards Prize in 1905 and by a Carnegie Institution grant from 1903–1905. Bryn Mawr was in the process of creating a research professorship for her when she died.

TO FIND OUT MORE . . .

- Ogilvie, Marilyn Bailey. *Women in Science.* Cambridge, MA: The MIT Press, 1986.

- Vare, Ethlie Ann, and Greg Ptacek. *Mothers of Invention: From the Bra to the Bomb.* New York: William Morrow, 1988.

Bertha Van Hoosen, 1863–1952

The surgeon and feminist Bertha Van Hoosen worked to better the lot of both her colleagues and her patients. She founded and served as the first president of the American Medical Women's Association. She was also a pioneer in the use of anesthesia during childbirth, which American doctors then considered unsafe. Although she was an accomplished surgeon, she devoted much of her career to women's health concerns.

Bertha, the younger of two daughters, was born on a farm in Stony Creek, Michigan. Her mother was a teacher and her father an uneducated Canadian who had made a comfortable sum digging gold in California. Bertha attended local public schools and then enrolled in the literature department at the University of Michigan, just as her sister had done. She decided to earn her M.D. from Michigan, partly for the independence a medical career offered, and worked her way through medical school when her father refused to bankroll her study.

After four years of medical school and four more of clinical residence, Van Hoosen opened her own private practice in Chicago in 1892. It was difficult at first to establish a clientele, but her competence soon overcame patients' misgivings about a woman doctor. She lectured on the side at Northwestern University for the five years it took to establish her practice, and was soon firmly established in Chicago medical circles.

When Northwestern's Woman's Medical School closed in 1902, she was appointed to the staff at the Illinois University Medical School, where she taught obstetrics and gynecology. This was a remarkable affirmation of her support in the community at a time when women physicians were still barred from membership in the Chicago Gynecological and Obstetrical Society. She taught there for a decade.

During her time at Illinois University,

Van Hoosen experimented with the injection of scopolamine and morphine during childbirth. The anesthesia killed the pain while allowing the patient to remain conscious, in a state known as "twilight sleep." In four years, she had delivered over two thousand healthy children using scopolamine-morphine injections, and considered the method to be "the greatest boon the Twentieth Century could give to women." Her work was controversial. Most doctors would not use this method of anesthesia during childbirth, while on the other side of the equation, some feminists demanded that it be considered a right of every woman to give birth without pain.

Van Hoosen was always involved in one way or another in women's issues in medicine. As a talented and demanding teacher, she was an inspiration to her women students, whom she called her "surgical daughters." She was also a very good surgeon who often performed operations for nonsurgical women physicians. In 1915 she became even more involved in women's issues when she founded the American Medical Women's Association. As president, she became one of the early feminists to demand the right of women to

> **Van Hoosen founded the American Medical Women's Association in 1915.**

serve in the military when she agitated to allow women physicians to serve during World War I. (They were not permitted to serve).

Bertha Van Hoosen's long and deeply committed career came to an end when she died at age eighty-nine. She had never had time for a family of her own, but stayed in touch with her parents (who supported her career after initially opposing it) and her widowed sister, Alice. Like many other women scientists of her time, her work was her primary love in life. She was an active surgeon nearly until her death and performed her last operation at age eighty-eight.

TO FIND OUT MORE ...

- Sicherman, Barbara, and Carol Hurd Green, eds. *Notable American Women: The Modern Period. A Biographical Dictionary.* Cambridge, MA: The Belknap Press of Harvard University Press, 1980.

- Van Hoosen, Bertha. *Petticoat Surgeon.* Chicago: Pellegrini & Cudahy, 1947.

Margaret Floy Washburn, 1871–1939

· ·

Margaret Washburn was a psychologist of extraordinarily high stature. She became the first woman president of the American Psychological Association (the second was elected fifty years later) and she was elected to the rarefied National Academy of Sciences. She excelled in every area of her scientific discipline: She published influential works, worked effectively in psychological associations, and was recognized for her work by her peers. What is more, she accomplished all this from Vassar College, a women's college with no graduate psychology department, where she was expected to undertake a heavy teaching and administrative load.

Washburn had early training for the unruffled persona she presented to her scientific peers. Her childhood in genteel 1870s Harlem and, later, in Walden, New York, left her with a strong sense of the importance of proper deportment. She enrolled at Vassar at fifteen and graduated with a dual interest in philosophy and science. Psychology appeared to her to combine the two, and so she took the bold step of presenting herself to the Columbia board of trustees as a candidate for admission.

The trustees allowed her to attend lectures at Columbia, but only as an auditor. Washburn transferred to Cornell University, where she earned a scholarship, had full graduate status, and became, in 1894, the first woman to receive a Ph.D. in psychology. Her excellent work, including a dissertation on the role visual perception plays in the judgment of distance and direction, earned her membership in the APA (American Psychological Association) on her graduation.

Washburn moved about from 1894 to 1904, taking positions at Wells College (1894–1900), Cornell (1900–1902), and the University of Cincinnati (1902–1903). Cincinnati made her head of its psychology department, but it was not considered a major research university and was too far away from home for Washburn. When Vassar had an opening for her in 1904 as an associate professor in psychology, she gladly took it.

Washburn had thirty-three enormously productive years at Vassar. She wrote an influential textbook, *The Animal Mind*, in 1908 and was promoted that same year to full professor. She maintained a rigorous schedule at Vassar while contributing to her discipline, serving on the APA's influential council from 1912 to 1914, as its president in 1921, and as the co-editor of the American Journal of Psychology from 1925 onward.

> *Washburn preempted any possible criticism relating to her gender by being an extremely methodical researcher.*

Her single-minded approach to her profession meant that she was an excellent but somewhat reserved lecturer—she needed to devote as much personal time as possible to her research and outside activities in order to achieve in her profession. Washburn preempted any possible criticism relating to her gender by being an extremely methodical researcher. She once pointed out, in her own wry way, "I smile to reflect what comments upon the feminine mind I should have made if I were a man and my contributors [to the AJP] women."

Margaret Washburn suffered a debilitating stroke at Vassar in 1937. She died two years later at home in Poughkeepsie, New York.

TO FIND OUT MORE . . .

- O'Connell, Agnes N., and Nancy Felipe Russo. *Models of Achievement: Reflections of Eminent Women in Psychology.*

    - Ogilvie, Marilyn Bailey. *Women in Science.* Cambridge, MA: The MIT Press, 1986.

- Scarborough, Elizabeth, and Laurel Furumoto. *Untold Lives: The First Generation of American Women Psychologists.* New York: Columbia University Press, 1987.

Anna Johnson Pell Wheeler, 1883–1966

$\cdot \quad \cdot$

Anna Wheeler was a mathematician at a time when women mathematicians were extremely rare. After extensive study (she eventually earned a Ph.D. and two master's degrees in mathematics), she was unable to find a permanent teaching position until her husband, also a mathematician, suffered a stroke and needed to be replaced.

Anna Johnson was born in Calliope, Iowa, to Swedish immigrants, Amelia and Andrew Johnson. Her father supported the family as a furniture dealer and undertaker. Anna was a quick, shy student; she graduated from Akron High School at age sixteen and earned her B.A. from the University of South Dakota at twenty.

Her mathematical mentor at the University was Sergei Degaev, a former Russian double agent who fled Russia when both his revolutionary cohorts and the government turned against him. He renamed himself Alexander Pell and moved to the United States. As Anna Johnson's professor, he encouraged her to pursue higher education. She earned two master's degrees, one from Radcliffe and another from the University of Iowa, and in 1906 won a Wellesley fellowship to study in Germany at Göttingen University under David Hilbert.

She jumped at the opportunity and, indeed, excelled at Göttingen, where she wrote a Ph.D. thesis. In 1907 Pell joined her in Germany, and the two were married. Anna Pell was twenty-four. Her work with David Hilbert took a nasty turn when they clashed over the thesis, and the Pells returned to South Dakota without her degree. When a teaching position opened up for Alexander Pell in Chicago, however, Anna Pell was able to earn a Ph.D. from the University of Chicago on the strength of her work in Germany.

No teaching jobs were available at Chicago for her until her husband suffered a debilitating stroke in 1911. She took over his work for the rest of the year, but in 1912 moved her invalid husband to the women's college Mount Holyoke, where she had a more secure teaching and research position. In 1918 she moved to another women's college, Bryn Mawr, where she became the head of the mathematics department. She spent most of the next thirty years there, until her retirement in 1948.

In 1921 Pell died. Anna Pell remarried in 1925, but her second husband, Mount Holyoke classics scholar Arthur Wheeler, also died of a stroke in 1932. Anna Wheeler resumed her work, which focused on linear algebra of infinitely many variables, with renewed intensity. In 1933 she extended a helping hand to another woman mathematician, **Emmy Noether**, a Jewish algebraist fleeing Nazi Germany. In 1940 she was honored by the Women's Centennial Congress as one of one hundred women who excelled in fields inaccessible to women a century before.

Wheeler retired at age sixty-five, but remained healthy until her sudden death at eighty-two.

> *She earned two master's degrees, one from Radcliffe and another from the University of Iowa, and in 1906 won a Wellesley fellowship to study in Germany at Göttingen University under David Hilbert.*

TO FIND OUT MORE . . .

- Ogilvie, Marilyn Bailey. *Women in Science.* Cambridge, MA: The MIT Press, 1986.

Anna Wessels Williams, 1863–1954

Bacteriologist Anna Wessels Williams was the first researcher to isolate a strain of the diptheria bacillus that was particularly useful in the production of an antitoxin for the disease. She was also the first scientist to observe the bodies indicative of rabies in the brain tissue of infected animals. Yet these discoveries were named, respectively, the "Park 8" strain and "Negri bodies," after the male researchers who received credit for the discoveries.

Williams was twenty-four when her sister Millie nearly died from eclampsia, a toxemia of pregnancy. Her baby was stillborn. Williams, spurred by a desire to learn how to change such tragic endings, enrolled at the Women's Medical College of the New York Infirmary. Her obstetrics and gynecology professor there was **Elizabeth Blackwell**, the first American woman awarded a medical degree. After graduation, she soon realized that the practice of medicine was too frustrating for her; there

were too many diseases without effective treatments, and as a doctor she could do little but prescribe whatever was available. In 1894 she accepted a position as an assistant bacteriologist in the diagnostic laboratory of the New York City Department of Health, run by William Hallock Park.

Diphtheria was then a difficult disease to treat; the antitoxin was difficult to produce, and the death rate in New York City was shooting up dramatically. In her first year at the laboratory, Williams isolated a strain of *Corynebacterium diphtheriae* that efficiently produced plenty of toxin. The discovery was instrumental in New York's pioneering antidiphtheria campaign; it made it possible for antitoxin to be produced in larger quantities. In a widely copied program, the city distributed antitoxin for free to those who could not pay. The credit for the discovery went to the lab director, William Park, although he was on vacation when Williams isolated the strain.

Williams continued on at Parks's laboratory, doing research on the causes of measles, smallpox, and rabies. In 1896 she brought a culture of rabies virus to the United States from the Pasteur Institute in Paris. By 1898 the culture had made large-scale vaccine production possible. Williams spent several years looking for ways to diagnose rabies quickly; when she started at the laboratory, rabies was diagnosed by injecting rabbits with the brain tissue of the dog suspected to be rabies. If the rabbit developed rabies, any patient bitten by the dog could be supposed to have rabies. By the time the rabbit developed the disease, however, the patient was likely to have become dangerously ill.

Her research was instrumental in the development of a diptheria antitoxin.

In her research, Williams had noted the presence of a distinctive type of cell in smears of brain tissue from rabid animals. She was still backing up her hypothesis that these "bodies" were diagnostic of rabies when, in 1904, the Italian researcher Adelchi Negri published his findings on what would thereafter be called "Negri bodies." Williams responded by publishing her superior method of staining and preparing brain tissue to detect the bodies. Her contribution shortened the process of diagnosing rabies further, from several days to within half an hour.

Williams published prolifically and was well respected within her field, despite the names given her discoveries. She never ascended past the post of assistant director at the New York laboratory, however, and was forced by regulations to retire at age seventy despite petitions from coworkers to Mayor Laguardia. It was certainly a loss to New York bacteriology; Williams lived for twenty more years in retirement with her sister in Westwood, New Jersey. She was ninety years old when she died.

TO FIND OUT MORE . . .

- O'Hern, Elizabeth Moot. *Profiles of Pioneer Women Scientists.* Washington, D.C.: Acropolis Books, Ltd., 1986.

- Sicherman, Barbara, and Carol Hurd Green, eds. *Notable American Women: The Modern Period. A Biographical Dictionary.* Cambridge, MA: The Belknap Press of Harvard University Press, 1980.

- Vare, Ethlie Ann, and Greg Ptacek. *Mothers of Invention: From the Bra to the Bomb, Forgotten Women and their Unforgettable Ideas.* New York: William Morrow and Company, Inc., 1988.

- Williams' papers are at the Schlesinger Library at Radcliffe College.

Mary Sophie Young, 1872–1919

When Mary Sophie Young died prematurely at the age of forty-seven, Texas lost a dedicated botanist. She came late to her profession, but in nine short years she succeeded in trading and collecting thousands of plants for the University of Texas herbarium, of which she served as curator.

Born in Glendale, Ohio, of educated parents, Young was given a rigorous education from the age of four, and proved a shy, diligent student. When, as a child, she followed her older brothers on rambles in the surrounding country, she learned to keep up uncomplainingly despite her smaller size. Much later, when she was tramping determinedly through the Texas mountains, she showed the same perseverance.

After earning her bachelor's degree at Wellesley College near Boston, Massachusetts, she spent thirteen years (1895–1908) as a schoolteacher in Kansas City, Kansas; Dundee, Illinois; Fond-du-Lac, Wisconsin; and Sullivan, Missouri. At the same time, however, she enrolled whenever possible in summer and correspondence courses. After a much-interrupted period of hard work, she earned her Ph.D. in 1910 from the University of Chicago.

The University of Texas at Austin hired Young on her graduation as a tutor in botany. She was promoted to instructor after a year and to the position of curator of the university's herbarium after another year. Her teaching experience served her well in classes; she taught freshmen botany and taxonomy and took her better students with her on collecting trips. As the curator of the herbarium, she collected thousands of specimens herself and traded thousands more with other herbaria all over the country.

Young took several long collecting trips around Texas from 1912 to 1918, but she recorded one trip—in 1914—in humorous detail in a daily journal. She usually traveled with a gun, even on short trips, to protect herself in the lonely Texas wilds, but she seldom used it on anything but rabbits. On her 1914 trip to the Trans-Pecos area of western Texas, Young also brought along a seventeen-year-old student, Carey Tharp, for company and added protection.

Her funds were limited to the small amount she could eke out of the University, supplemented with her own meager earnings. Young bought a buggy and two burros (Balaam and Nebuchadnezzar) for a grand total of seventeen dollars. Soon, however, she found that the lack of money was far less pressing than the general shortage of food. Beans, bacon, wormy cornmeal and flour for biscuits and hardtack were supplemented by jack rabbits shot with Young's gun, but she wrote in her journal that "jack rabbit meat would make good sole leather." Food, or rather the lack of it, preoccupied her for much of the trip.

Young spent six weeks traveling hundreds of miles into the mountains. Carey helped her to dry specimens, and she helped him with the math problems he'd brought along. By the end of the trip, her shoes had worn out and the burros could only be moved by force. Young described

Armed with her gun and her notes, Young tramped the Texas mountains to bring back new specimens for the University of Texas at Austin's herbarium.

choking Nebuchadnezzar repeatedly by covering his nostrils in order to get him moving on one particularly bad day. They endured a plague of caterpillars, torrential rain, "very large and very hungry" mosquitoes, and rattlesnake scares to bring back several hundred new specimens of Texas flora.

Young took other trips into new areas of Texas, sometimes employing other students like Carey, but she never recorded another in the same way as she had the 1914 trip. She published a definitive guide to plants of the region, *A Key to the Families and Genera of Flowering Plants and Ferns in the Vicinity of Austin, Texas*, in 1917. Two years later, when she was in the hospital for a routine operation, a surgeon found her body riddled with cancer. She died within a month, leaving much work yet undone; still, in her nine short years as a botanist, she had made an impressive contribution to the state's botanical research.

TO FIND OUT MORE ...

- Bonta, Margaret Meyers. *Women in the Field: America's Pioneering Naturalists*. College Station, TX: Texas A&M University Press, 1991.

- Young's papers are at the Eugene T. Barker Texas history Center at the University of Texas, Austin.

Index by Occupation

Anthropologists
Ruth Fulton Benedict
Elsie Clews Parsons
Hortense Powdermaker
Ellen Churchill Semple

Archaeologists
Hetty Goldman
Harriet Boyd Hawes

Astronomers
Annie Jump Cannon
Henrietta Swan Leavitt
Antonia Caetania Maury
Cecilia Payne-Gaposchkin

Bacteriologists
Hattie Elizabeth Alexander
Sara Elizabeth Branham
Cornelia Mitchell Downs
Alice Catherine Evans
Alice Hamilton
Elizabeth McCoy
Anna Wessels Williams

Biochemists
Gerty Theresa Radnitz Cori
Jane Ane Russell

Biologists
Rachel Carson
Helen Dean King
Nettie Maria Stevens

Botanists
Annie Montague Alexander
Emma Lucy Braun
Mary Agnes Meara Chase
Caroline Dorman
Alice Eastwood
Margaret Clay Ferguson
Ynes Mexia
Mary Sophie Young

Cancer researchers
May Edward Chinn
Virginia Kneeland Frantz
Maud Caroline Slye

Chemists
Emma Perry Carr
Mary Engle Pennington
Florence Barbara Seibert

Conservationists
Rachel Carson
Caroline Dorman
Ann Haven Morgan

Cytologists
Alice Middleton Boring
Ethel Browne Harvey
Nettie Maria Stevens

Entomologist
Edith Patch

Engineers
Edith Clarke (electrical)
Irmgard Flügge-Lotz (aeronautical)
Lillian Evelyn Moller Gilbreth (industrial)

Faith healer
Aimee Semple McPherson

Geneticists
Alice Middleton Boring
Barbara McClintock
Nettie Maria Stevens

Geologists
Florence Bascom
Julia Anna Gardner

Gynecologists
Sophia Josephine Kleegman
Lena Levine
Anita Newcomb McGee

Home economists
Lillian Evelyn Moller Gilbreth
Flemmie Kittrell

Inventors
Katherine Burr Blodgett
Bette Nesmith Graham
Ida Cohen Rosenthal

Mathematicians
Hilda Geiringer
Anna Johnson Pell Wheeler

Microbiologists
Gladys Rowena Henry Dick
Elizabeth Lee Hazen
Rebecca Craighill Lancefield

Naturalist
Anna Botsford Comstock

Nurses

Florence Aby Blanchfield
Martha Minerva Franklin
Margaret Sanger
Mabel Staupers

Nutritionists

Grace Arabell Goldsmith
Flemmie Kittrell

Ornithologists

Annie Montague Alexander
Caroline Dorman
Amelia Rudolph Laskey
Margaret Morse Nice
Cordelia Stanwood

Paleontologists

Annie Montague Alexander
Tilly Edinger
Winifred Goldring

Pathologists

Alice Hamilton
Maud Caroline Slye

Pediatricians

Ethel Collins Dunham
Martha May Eliot

Physicians

Hattie Elizabeth Alexander
Sara Josephine Baker
Mary Elizabeth Bass
May Edward Chinn
Gladys Rowena Henry Dick
Grace Arabell Goldsmith
Sara Claudia Murray Jordan
Esther Clayson Pohl Lovejoy
Anita Newcomb McGee
Alice Woodby McKane
Susan La Flesche Picotte
Florence Rena Sabin
Ida Sophia Scudder

Physicists

Elda Emma Anderson
Katherine Burr Blodgett
Maria Gertrude Goeppert Mayer

Psychiatrists

Helen Flanders Dunbar
Frieda Fromm-Reichmann
Lillian Evelyn Moller Gilbreth
Karen Danielsen Horney
Lena Levine

Psychologists

Augusta Fox Bronner
Alice Isabel Bever Bryan
Mary Whiton Calkins

June Etta Downey
Else Frenkel-Brunswik
Florence Laura Goodenough
Leta Anna Stetter Hollingworth
Lillien Jane Martin
Carolyn Wood Sherif
Margaret Floy Washburn

Physiologist
Ida Henrietta Hyde

Sociologists
Elsie Clews Parsons
Hortense Powdermaker

Surgeons
Virginia Apgar
Matilda Arabella Evans
Virginia Kneeland Frantz
Bertha Van Hoosen

Zoologists
Alice Middleton Boring
Julia Anna Gardner
Libbie Henrietta Hyman
Ann Haven Morgan